Pressure Cooker Recipes for Beginners 2021

Easy And Delicious Dishes To Prepare At Home

Wanda Hastings

Sommario

Introduction

Considering the principle of diet in current times are based upon fasting, instead our keto instant pot is based upon the extreme decrease of carbs.
This kind of diet is based on the intake of specific foods that allow you to slim down faster permitting you to slim down approximately 3 kg each week.
You will certainly see how simple it will be to make these tasty meals with the tools available as well as you will certainly see that you will certainly be satisfied.
If you are reluctant concerning this fantastic diet plan you simply have to try it as well as analyze your results to a short time, trust me you will be pleased.
Bear in mind that the most effective method to reduce weight is to analyze your situation with the help of a specialist.

Lunch

Italian-Style Greens with Eggs and Cheese

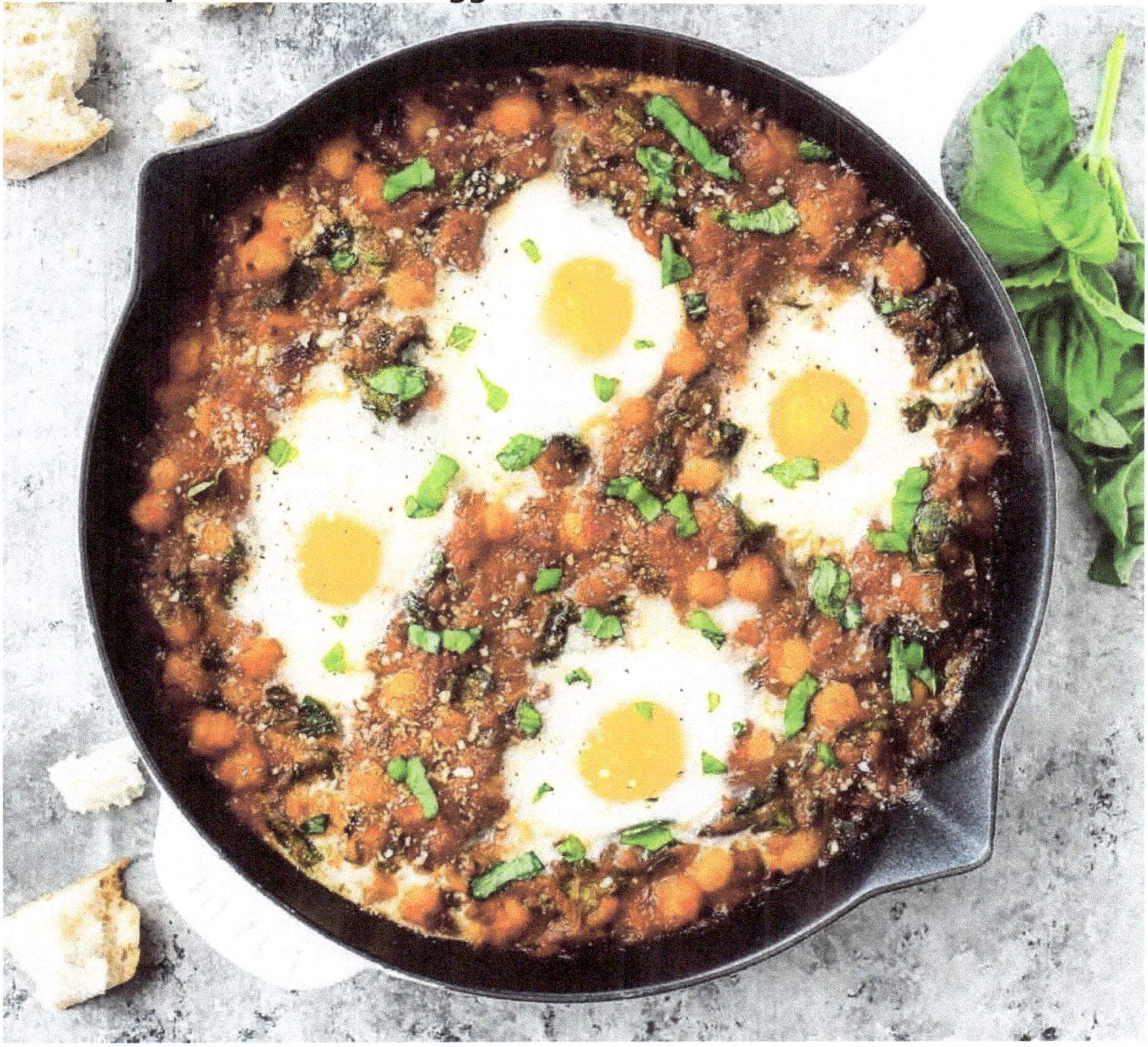

(Ready in about 10 minutes | Servings 4)

Per serving: 291 Calories; 19.8g Fat; 8.8g Carbs; 20.9g Protein; 1.8g Sugars

Ingredients

2 teaspoons butter, melted 6 eggs 2 tablespoons cream cheese Sea salt and ground black pepper, to taste 1/2 teaspoon paprika 1/2 teaspoon ground bay leaf 1 pound collard greens, torn into pieces 1 cup broth, preferably homemade 1 cup Provolone cheese, crumbled

Directions

Press the "Sauté" button to heat up your Instant Pot. Now, warm the butter. Whisk the eggs with cream cheese in a mixing dish. Once hot, add the egg/cheese mixture to the Instant Pot. Now, add the salt, black pepper, ground bay leaf and collard greens. Secure the lid. Choose "Manual" mode and Low pressure; cook for 3 minutes. Once cooking is complete, use a quick pressure release; carefully remove the lid. Add Provolone cheese on top and press the "Sauté" button again. Continue to cook until everything is heated through; serve warm. Bon appétit!

Mini Meatloaves with Cheese
(Ready in about 20 minutes | Servings 6)
Per serving: 276 Calories; 17.5g Fat; 3.3g Carbs; 25.6g Protein; 1.7g Sugars

Ingredients

1/2 pound ground pork 1/2 pound ground turkey 1/2 yellow onion, chopped 1/2 cup pork rinds, crushed 1 tablespoon coconut aminos 2 tablespoons fresh cilantro, chopped 3 eggs, whisked Sea salt and ground black pepper, to taste 1 teaspoon cayenne pepper 1/2 teaspoon dried dill weed 1/2 teaspoon oregano 1 tablespoon mint, chopped 1/2 cup pasta sauce, no sugar 1/2 cup cheddar cheese, grated

Directions

Mix all ingredients, except for pasta sauce and cheddar cheese, until everything is well incorporated. Now, add 1 cup of water and a metal trivet to the Instant Pot. Divide the mixture among muffin cups; top with pasta sauce. Lower the muffin cups onto the trivet. Secure the lid. Choose "Manual" mode and High pressure; cook for 6 minutes. Once cooking is complete, use a natural pressure release; carefully remove the lid. Top with the shredded cheese; cover with the lid and allow your muffins to sit in the residual heat for 4 to 7 minutes. Allow the muffins to stand for a few minutes before removing from the cups. Bon appétit!

Eggs with Green Cabbage

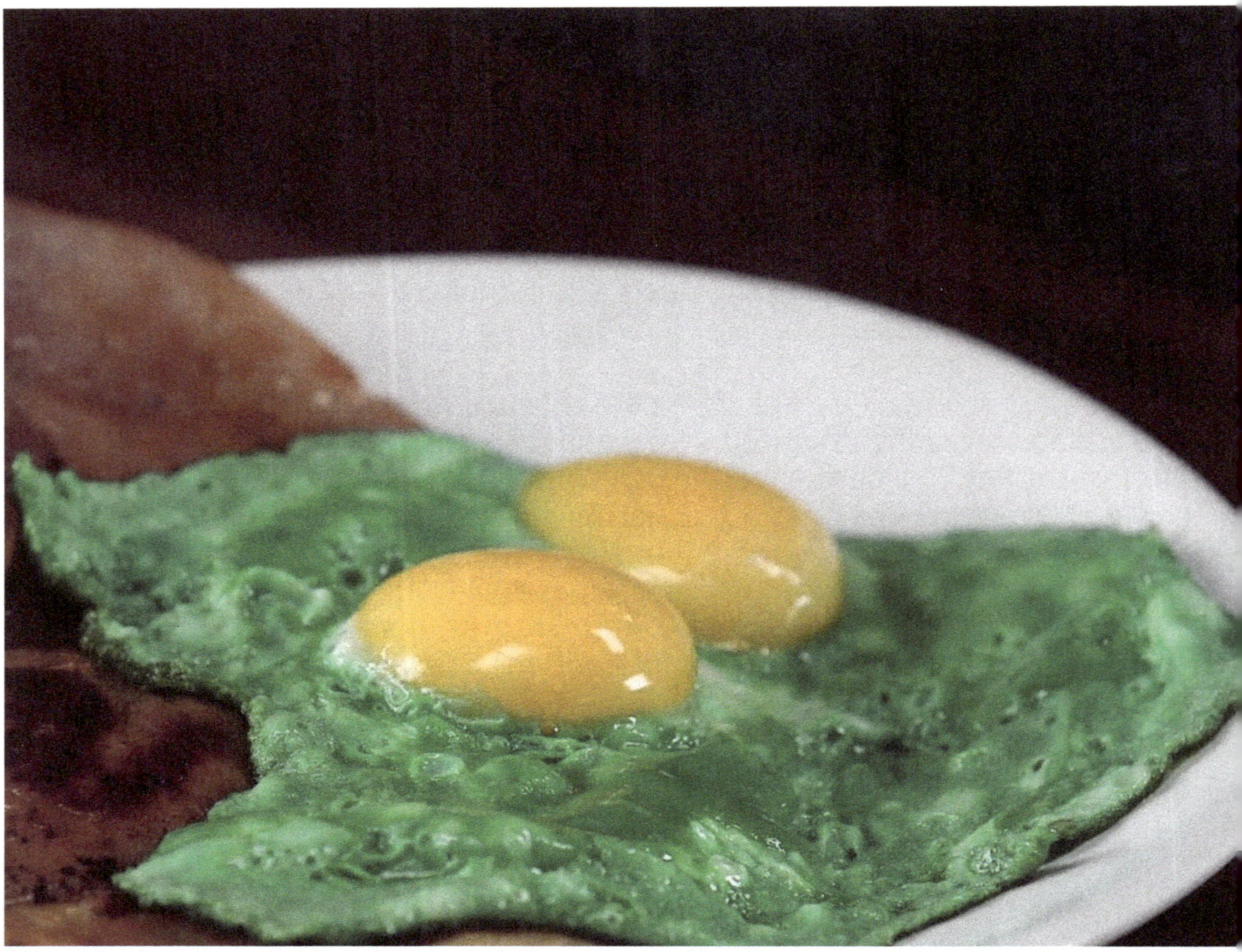

(Ready in about 10 minutes | Servings 4)

Per serving: 164 Calories; 11.2g Fat; 9.1g Carbs; 7.3g Protein; 4.9g Sugars

Ingredients

2 tablespoons olive oil 1 pound green cabbage, shredded 1 teaspoon garlic, smashed 4 eggs, whisked 1/2 teaspoon celery seeds 1/2 teaspoon mustard seeds 1/2 teaspoon dried parsley flakes 1/2 teaspoon red pepper flakes, crushed Sea salt and ground black pepper, to your liking 1 tablespoon Worcestershire sauce

Directions

Press the "Sauté" button to heat up your Instant Pot. Now, heat the olive oil until sizzling. Then, sauté green cabbage for 1 to 2 minutes. Add garlic and cook an additional 30 seconds. Add the remaining ingredients. Secure the lid. Choose "Manual" mode and Low pressure; cook for 3 minutes. Once cooking is complete, use a quick pressure release; carefully remove the lid. Divide the mixture between serving plates and serve warm. Bon appétit!

Garden Omelet with Colby Cheese
(Ready in about 15 minutes | Servings 4)
Per serving: 284 Calories; 24.2g Fat; 6g Carbs; 10.5g Protein; 2.4g Sugars
Ingredients
2 tablespoons olive oil 1 yellow onion, chopped 1 zucchini, sliced 2 garlic cloves, minced 4 eggs, beaten 4 tablespoons heavy whipped cream Sea salt and ground black pepper, to taste 1 teaspoon cayenne pepper 1 tablespoon Cajun seasoning 1/2 cup Colby cheese, shredded
Directions Press the "Sauté" button to heat up your Instant Pot. Heat the oil and sauté the onion until tender and translucent. Now, add zucchini and garlic and cook for 1 minute more. Thoroughly combine the eggs, heavy whipped cream, salt, black pepper, cayenne pepper, and Cajun seasoning. Add the egg mixture to the Instant Pot. Secure the lid. Choose "Manual" mode and High pressure; cook for 6 minutes. Once cooking is complete, use a quick pressure release; carefully remove the lid. Add shredded cheese and put the lid on the Instant Pot. Let it sit in the residual heat for 4 minutes. Serve warm and enjoy!

Weeknight Meat and Egg Muffins
(Ready in about 10 minutes | Servings 4)
Per serving: 438 Calories; 27.2g Fat; 4.5g Carbs; 42.2g Protein; 1.8g Sugars
Ingredients
2 teaspoons grapeseed oil 1/2 yellow onion, chopped 1 cup brown mushrooms, chopped 2 cloves garlic, smashed 1 teaspoon ground mustard 1 tablespoon coconut aminos Kosher salt and freshly ground black pepper, to taste 1 pound ground beef 2 eggs 1 cup Romano cheese, grated 1/2 teaspoon dried rosemary 1 teaspoon dried sage 1/2 teaspoon dried thyme 1/2 teaspoon garlic powder 1/2 cup tomato, purèed
Directions
Thoroughly combine all ingredients until everything is well combined. Then, add 1 cup of water and a metal trivet to the Instant Pot. Divide the mixture among muffin cups; lower the muffin cups onto the trivet. Secure the lid. Choose "Manual" mode and High pressure; cook for 6 minutes. Once cooking is complete, use a natural pressure release; carefully remove the lid. Serve warm.

Hoisin-Glazed Baby Back Ribs

Ingredients for 4-6 servings:

1 cup Hoisin Sauce ½ cup honey 1 tbsp Chinese five-spice powder 5 tbsp gochujang divided 2 tbsp minced fresh ginger 2 2 ½- to 3-lb racks baby back pork ribs each cut half if pressure cooking or cut into 3 or 4 rib sections if slow cooking 2 tbsp finely chopped fresh cilantro 2 tbsp sesame seeds toasted 3 scallions thinly sliced

Directions and total time – 1-2 h

• START: In a large bowl, whisk together the hoisin, honey, five-spice powder and 2 tbsp gochujang. Measure ¾ cup of the mixture into a small bowl and stir in the remaining 3 tbsp gochujang and the ginger; set aside at room temperature if pressure cooking or cover and refrigerate if slow cooking. Add the rib sections to the remaining hoisin mixture in the large bowl and turn to coat. Place the steam rack in a 6-quart Instant Pot, then pour in 1 cup water. Arrange the ribs upright in a circle, with the meaty sides facing the walls of the pot. • Fast (Pressure Cook): Lock the lid in place and move the pressure valve to Sealing. Select Pressure Cook or Manual; make sure the pressure level is set to High. Set the cooking time for 25 minutes. When pressure cooking is complete, allow the pressure to reduce naturally for 15 minutes, then release the remaining steam by moving the pressure valve to Venting. Press Cancel, then carefully open the pot. Let cool for 5 minutes. -ORSlow (Slow cooking): Select More/High Sauté and bring the water to a boil. Press Cancel, lock the lid in place and move the pressure valve to Venting. Select Slow Cook and set the temperature to More/High. Set the cooking time for 8 to 9 hours; the ribs are done when a skewer inserted into the meat between the bones meets no resistance. Press Cancel, then carefully open the pot. Let cool for 5 minutes. • FINISH: While the ribs cool, heat the broiler with a rack about 6 inches from the element. Line a rimmed baking sheet with foil. Using tongs, carefully transfer the ribs meat side up to the prepared baking sheet. Generously brush with half of the reserved hoisin mixture and broil until the glaze begins to bubble, 2 to 3 minutes. Remove from the broiler, brush with the remaining mixture and continue to broil until bubbling, another 2 to 3 minutes. Cool for 5 minutes, then cut between the bones to separate into individual ribs. Transfer to a platter, then sprinkle with the cilantro, sesame seeds and scallions.

Awesome Slow Cooker Pot Roast
Ingredients for 12 servings:
2 (10.75 ounce) cans condensed cream of mushroom soup 1 (1 ounce) package dry onion soup mix 1 ¼ cups water 5 ½ pounds pot roast
Directions and total time – 8 hrs
• In a slow cooker, mix cream of mushroom soup, dry onion soup mix and water. Place pot roast in slow cooker and coat with soup mixture. • Cook on High setting for 3 to 4 hours, or on Low setting for 8 to 9 hours. Parmesan Roast Chicken with Lemon Ingredients for 6 servings: 2 lemons small 3 tsp kosher salt plus more to taste 3 tsp black pepper 2 tsp rosemary chopped 6 rosemary sprigs 2 tsp red pepper flakes plus more for serving, optional 1 whole chicken about 3 pounds extra-virgin olive oil for drizzling ⅓ cup parmesan finely grated 4 cups chicken stock Directions and total time – 30-60 m • Finely grate 2 teaspoons of zest from the lemons and place into a small bowl. (Save the zested lemon for the drippings.) • Stir in 3 teaspoons salt, pepper, chopped rosemary and red-pepper flakes (if using). Season the chicken inside and out with salt mixture and set aside. Stuff cavity of chicken with 2 rosemary springs. • Place the chicken breast-side down, add the chicken, the stock, and 2 of the rosemary springs into the inner pot. Place the inner pot into your Instant Pot and select Pressure Cook, and set to High pressure for 20 minutes. • When pressure cooking is complete, Quick Release the pressure. • Remove the lid, using tongs take the chicken out of the inner pot and drain the water. • Making sure that your inner pot is dry, place the air fryer basket (or trivet) into the pot, drizzle the chicken with the olive oil and place it into the basket. • Using the Air fryer Lid select Roast at 400°F for 25 minutes. In the middle of the cooking process sprinkle the chicken with the parmesan cheese. Continue roasting. • When cooking is complete the internal temperature should reach 165°F. Let the chicken rest for 5 to 10 minutes then squeeze juice from one of the zested lemons over the chicken. • Carve and serve drippings spooned over the meat.

Coconut-Curry Rice and Vegetable
Ingredients for 6 servings:
⅔ cup uncooked brown rice rinsed and drained 1 cup Water 1 tsp curry powder ¾ tsp salt divided 1 cup chopped green onion both green and white parts 1 cup sliced red or yellow bell pepper 1 cup matchstick carrots 1 cup chopped red or purple cabbage 1 can sliced water chestnuts drained, 8 oz 1 can no salt added chickpeas rinsed and drained, 15 oz 1 can lite coconut milk 13 oz 1 tbsp grated fresh ginger 1 ½ tbsp sugar
Directions and total time – 30-60 m
• Combine the rice, water, curry powder, and ¼ tsp of the salt in the Instant Pot. • Seal the lid, close the valve, and set the Manual/Pressure Cook button to 15 minutes. • Use a natural pressure release for about 12 minutes. When the valve drops, carefully remove the lid and stir in the remaining ingredients. • Press the Cancel button and set to Sauté. Then press the Adjust button to "More" or "High." Bring to a boil and boil for 2 minutes, or until all the ingredients are heated through, stirring occasionally.

Easy Chicken Noodle Soup

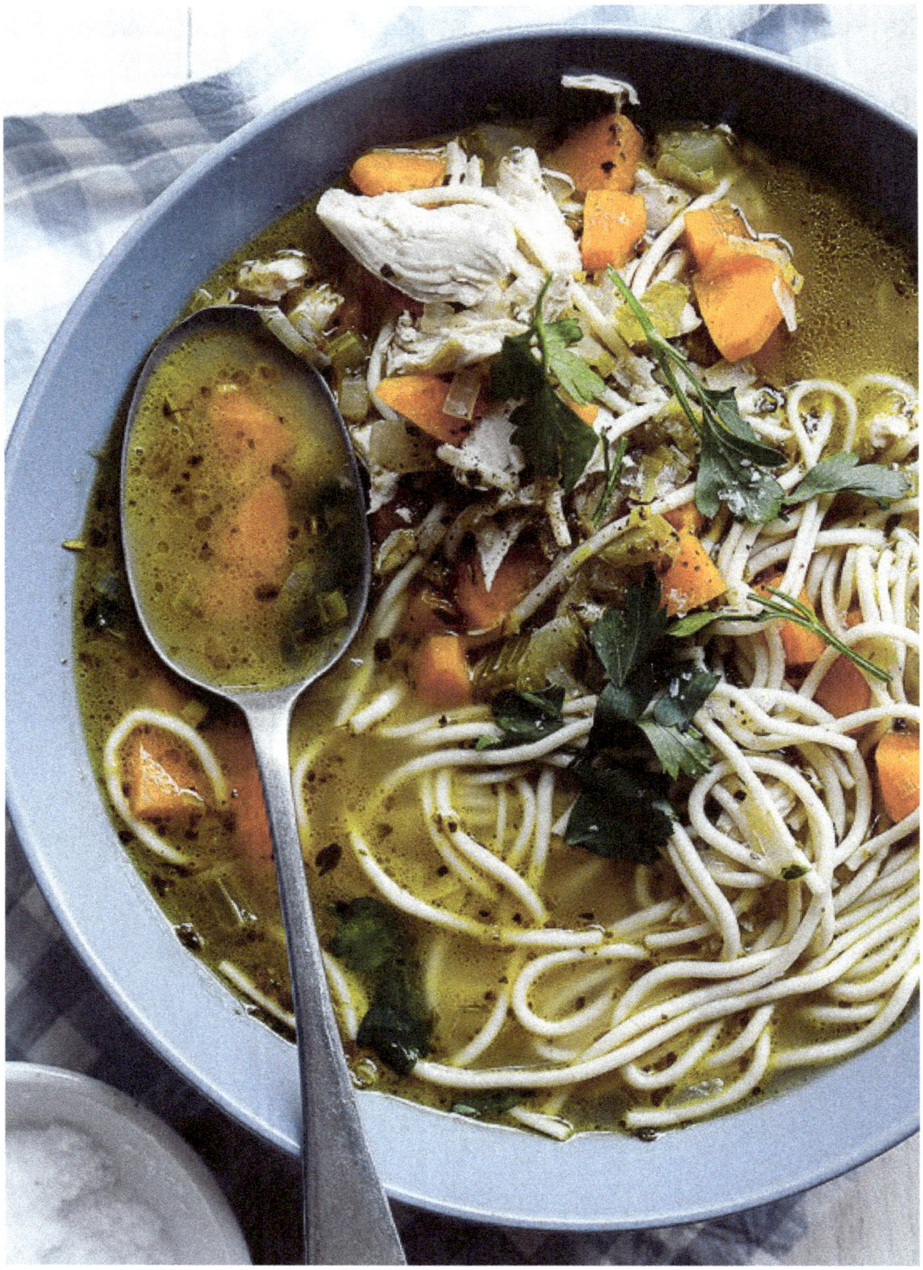

Ingredients for 4 servings:

½ lbs boneless skinless chicken breasts 1 carrot peeled and chopped (about ½ cup) 1 stalk celery sliced (about ½ cup) 2 oz uncooked extrawide egg noodles about 1 cup dry 4 cups Chicken Broth

Directions and total time – 30-60 m

• Season the chicken with salt and pepper. Add the carrot, celery, chicken, noodles and broth to a 6 quart Instant Pot. • Lock the lid and close the pressure release valve. Pressure cook on High pressure, setting the timer to 5 minutes (timer will begin counting down once pressure is reached- it takes about 15 minutes). When done, press Cancel and use the quick release method to release the pressure. • Remove the chicken from the pot. Shred the chicken and return to the pot. Season to taste.

Bean and Sausage Soup

Ingredients for 6 servings: 2 tbsp olive oil ½ lbs Italian-style chicken sausage casing removed 1 extra large onion diced (about 1 ½ cups) 2 cloves garlic minced 1 can white cannellini beans rinsed and drained, about 15 ounces 1 tsp Italian seasoning 4 cups Chicken Broth 3 cups packed finely chopped kale leaves trim leaves from stems before chopping 2 tbsp grated parmesan cheese

Directions and total time – 30-60 m • On a 6 quart Instant Pot, select the Saute setting. Heat the oil. Add the sausage and cook for 10 minutes or until well browned, stirring often to separate meat. Press Cancel. • Add the onion, garlic, beans, Italian seasoning and broth. Lock the lid and close the pressure release valve. Pressure cook on High pressure, setting the timer to 3 minutes (timer will begin counting down once pressure is reached- it takes about 10 minutes). When done, press Cancel and use the quick release method to release the pressure. • Stir in the kale and let stand for 5 minutes. Season to taste and sprinkle with the cheese.

Mongolian Beef
Ingredients for 6 servings:
1 ½ pounds flank or sirloin steak thinly sliced 2 tbsp corn starch 2 tbsp oil 1 cup Water ⅓ cup packed brown sugar ¾ cup reduced-sodium soy sauce 1 package spices for meat to taste 2 green onions cut into 1 inch pieces, green parts only
Directions and total time – 15-30 m • Place beef in large resealable bag. Add corn starch; close bag tightly and shake to coat beef. Heat oil in Instant Pot on SAUTÉ setting. Add beef to pot; cook and stir 3 minutes. Remove beef from pot. Add water; stirring with whisk to remove browned bits from bottom of pot. Stir in brown sugar, soy sauce and Seasoning Mix until well blended. Return beef to pot. Close lid. Set Valve to Seal. • Select PRESSURE COOK (MANUAL); cook 7 minutes on HIGH PRESSURE. When done, quick-release pressure. Open lid once pressure inside pot is completely released. (Check manufacturer's manual for safe operating instructions.) Stir in green onions.

Beef Stroganoff
Ingredients for 6 servings:
1 large onion diced (about 1 cup) 1 ¼ lbs boneless beef sirloin steak cut into thin strips 1 tsp paprika ½ tsp garlic powder 4 cups uncooked extra-wide egg noodles 2 cups water 2 tsp Worcestershire sauce 1 can Condensed Cream 10 ½ ounces ¼ cup sour cream 2 tbsp chopped fresh parsley
Directions and total time – 30-60 m • Season the beef with salt and pepper. Layer the onion, beef, paprika, garlic powder and noodles in a 6 quart Instant Pot. Pour the broth and Worcestershire over the noodles and spoon the soup on top (the order is important, so don't stir until after the cooking is done). • Lock the lid and close the pressure release valve. Pressure cook on High pressure, setting the timer to 8 minutes (timer will begin counting down once pressure is reached- it takes about 15 minutes). When done, press Cancel and use the quick release method to release the pressure. • Stir in the sour cream and let stand for 5 minutes uncovered. Season to taste and sprinkle with the parsley before serving.

Rigatoni & Tomatoes and Pancetta
Ingredients for 4-6 servings:
4 oz pancetta chopped fine 1 onion chopped fine ¼ tsp table salt 3 garlic cloves minced 2 anchovy fillets rinsed, patted dry, and minced 2 tsp fennel seeds lightly cracked ¼ tsp red pepper flakes 1 can diced tomatoes 28 ounce 2 cups chicken broth 1 ½ cups Water 1 lb rigatoni ¼ cup grated Pecorino Romano cheese plus extra for serving 2 tbsp minced fresh parsley
Directions and total time – 30-60 m • Using highest sauté function, cook pancetta in Instant Pot, stirring often, until browned and fat is well rendered, 6 to 10 minutes. Using slotted spoon, transfer pancetta to paper towel- lined plate; set aside for serving. • Add onion and salt to fat left in pot and cook, using highest sauté function, until onion is softened, about 5 minutes. Stir in garlic, anchovies, fennel seeds, and pepper flakes and cook until fragrant, about 1 minute. Stir in tomatoes and their juice, broth, and water, scraping up any browned bits, then stir in pasta. • Lock lid in place and close pressure release valve. Select Pressure Cook function on High and cook for 5 minutes. Turn off Instant Pot and quick-release pressure. Carefully remove lid, allowing steam to escape away from you. • Stir in Pecorino and season with salt and pepper to taste. Transfer to serving dish and let sit until sauce thickens slightly, about 5 minutes. Sprinkle with parsley and reserved pancetta. Serve, passing extra Pecorino separately.

Falafel in Pita Pockets

Ingredients for 4 servings:

1 cup dried chickpeas 4 cups Water 1 tsp fine sea salt 1 tbsp extra-virgin olive oil ½ tsp cumin ½ tsp coriander ½ tsp onion powder ¼ tsp garlic powder ¼ tsp fine sea salt ¼ tsp freshly ground black pepper 4 Persian cucumbers sliced 1 head romaine lettuce shredded 2 tomatoes thinly sliced ½ small red onion thinly sliced 6 whole-wheat pitas warmed and split ¾ cup tahini dressing for serving Harissa zhoug, or sambal oelek, for serving (optional)

Directions and total time – more than 2 h

• Combine the chickpeas, water, and salt in the Instant Pot and stir to dissolve the salt. Secure the lid and set the Pressure Release to Sealing. Select the Bean/Chili, Pressure Cook, or Manual and set the cooking time for 15 minutes at high pressure. Next, select the Timer or Delay function and set the time delay for 10 to 12 hours. (When the soaking time is complete, the pot will take about 10 minutes to come up to pressure before the cooking program begins.) • When the cooking program ends, let the pressure release for at least 15 minutes, then move the Pressure Release to Venting to release any remaining steam. Open the pot and, wearing heat-resistant mitts, lift out the inner pot and drain the chickpeas in a colander, then transfer them to a medium bowl. • Add 1 ½ tsps of the oil, the cumin, coriander, onion powder, garlic powder, salt, and pepper and toss to coat the chickpeas evenly with the oil and spices. • Heat the remaining 1 ½ tsp oil in a skillet over medium-high heat. Add the chickpeas and sauté. for 8 to 10 minutes, until the chickpeas are slightly browned and the spices are aromatic and toasted but not burned. Remove from the heat. • Tuck the cucumbers, lettuce, tomatoes, and onion into the pitas, then spoon ½ cup of the warm chickpeas into each pocket. Drizzle each filled pita with 2 tbsp tahini dressing and with hot sauce to taste. Serve the pita pockets while the chickpeas are warm.

Lettuce Wraps

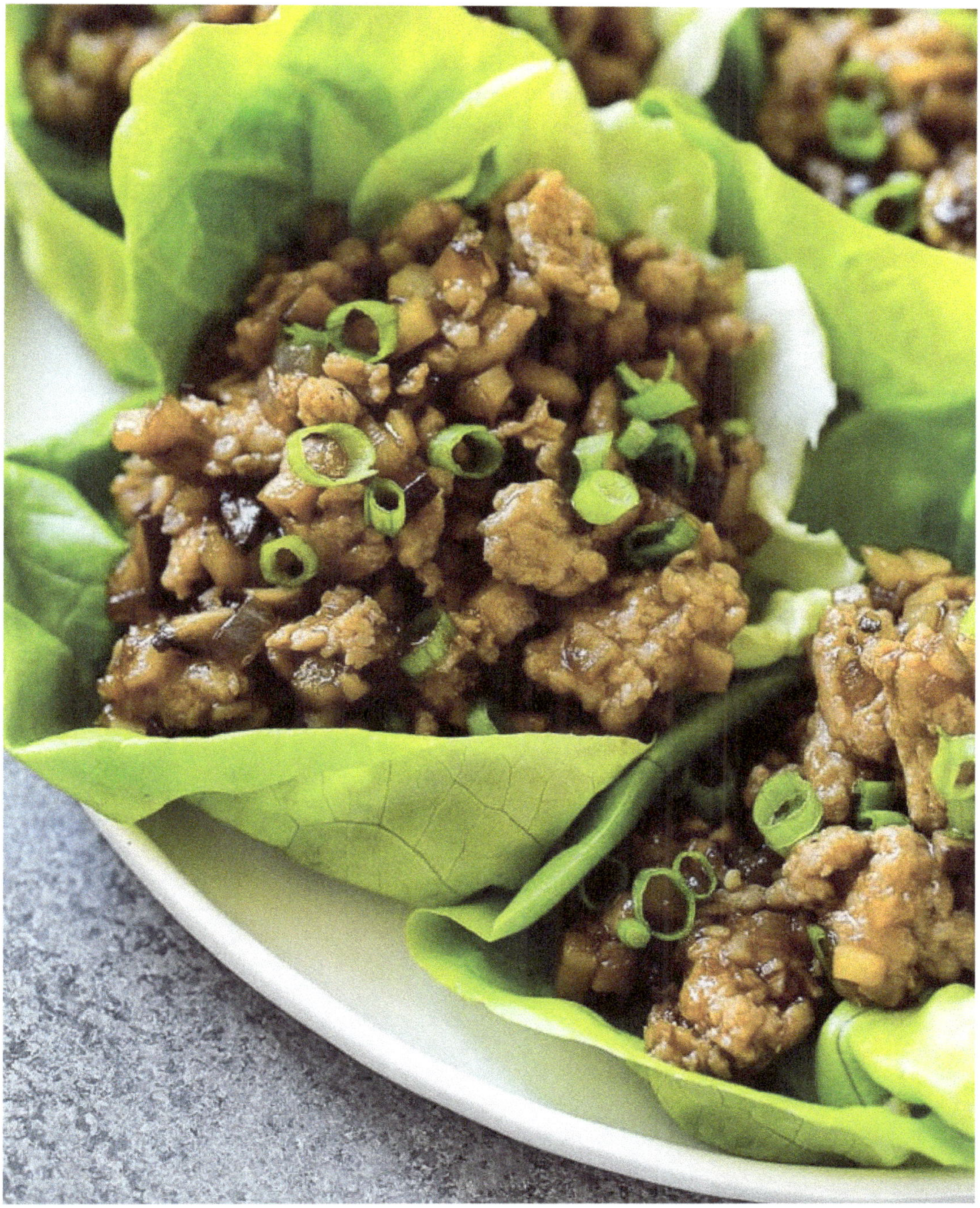

Ingredients for 4 servings:

2 tablespoons olive oil 1 lb ground pork 2 medium carrots diced 1 bunch green onions sliced ½ cup Water 1 cup Hoisin Sauce 1 cup soy sauce 2 tsp minced ginger ½ tsp red pepper flakes 8 oz water chestnuts can, drained 1 small head bib lettuce

Directions and total time – 15-30 m

• Press Sauté button on Instant Pot. Add oil, ground pork, carrots, and green onions to Instant Pot. Cook, stirring occasionally, 5 minutes. • Pour in water and deglaze bottom of pot. Turn Instant Pot off. • In a small bowl, mix hoisin sauce, soy sauce, ginger, and red pepper flakes together. Pour sauce and water chestnuts over pork. Do not stir. • Close lid and set pressure release to Sealing. • Press Manual or Pressure Cook button and adjust time to 2 minutes. • When the timer beeps, allow pressure to release naturally and then unlock lid and remove it. • Mix ingredients together. Scoop pork into bib lettuce leaves and serve.

Buffalo Wings
Ingredients for 4 servings:
2 pounds frozen chicken wings ½ tablespoon Cajun seasoning 1 ½ cups Water 1 cup buffalo wing sauce
Directions and total time – 15-30 m
• In a large bowl, toss chicken wings in Cajun seasoning so they are evenly coated. • Pour water into Instant Pot and add a trivet. • Place wings in a (7 inch) spring form pan. Create a foil sling and lower pan into Instant Pot. • Close lid and set pressure release to Sealing. • Press Manual or Pressure Cook button and adjust time to 15 minutes. • When the timer beeps, allow pressure to release naturally and then unlock lid and remove it. Remove pan from Instant Pot using foil sling. • Remove wings and brush with buffalo sauce. Serve hot.

BBQ Brisket Sandwiches
Ingredients for 6 servings:
1 cup Water 3 lb beef brisket cut into ½ lb chunks 1 tbsp smoked paprika ½ cup BBQ sauce 6 sesame seed buns toasted Additional toppings like sliced onion or pickles optional
Directions and total time – 1-2 h
• Pour one cup of water in the Instant Pot, followed by the brisket pieces. Sprinkle with smoked paprika. • Secure the lid, making sure the vent is closed. • Using the display panel select the MANUAL function. Use the +/- keys and program the Instant Pot for 60 minutes. • When the time is up, let the pressure naturally release for 15 minutes, then quick-release the remaining pressure. • Carefully remove the meat from the pot to a shallow dish and chop. • Stir in bbq sauce and ¼ cup - ½ cup of cooking juices to reach desired consistency. • Pile on toasted sesame seed buns and garnish as desired.

Pot Pie

Ingredients for 4 servings:

For the Stew: 2 cups broth of any sort 1 tbsp Worcestershire sauce 1 lb frozen ground meat. Choose from beef, buffalo, venison, pork, turkey, chicken, or even sausage meat—or a combo of any two you prefer. 2 tsp dried seasoning blend. Choose either a prepared seasoning such as Italian or Tex-Mex or a blend you create (rosemary, oregano, thyme, parsley, and basil are the norms, but enhance them with a little ground allspice or grated nutmeg). ½ tsp table salt optional ½ tsp ground black pepper 1 lb frozen unseasoned mixed vegetables. (4-5 cups) Choose from any unseasoned blend, so long as you omit any flavoring packets. Or use a combination of frozen corn kernels, bell pepper strips, chopped onion, and/or sliced carrots. ½ cup heavy or light cream but not "fat-free" cream 2 ½ tbsp all-purpose flour For the Biscuit Topping: 1 ¼ cups all-purpose flour 1 ½ tsp baking powder ½ tsp table salt 6 tbsp whole or low-fat milk 1 tbsp butter melted and cooled; or 1 tbsp oil of any sort you prefer 1 large egg 4 oz shredded semi-firm cheese. (1 cup) such as Cheddar, Swiss, or even a prepared blend, optional. ½ tsp mild paprika

Directions and total time – 30-60 m

• To make the stew, pour the broth and Worcestershire sauce into an Instant Pot. Set the pot's rack (with the handles up) or a large, open vegetable steamer inside the pot. Set the ground meat on the rack or in the steamer. Sprinkle the seasoning blend, salt (if using), and pepper over the meat. Lock the lid onto the pot. • Option 1 Max Pressure Cooker Press Pressure cook on Max Pressure for 18 minutes with the Keep Warm setting off and the valve closed. Option 2 All Pressure Cookers Press Meat/Stew or Pressure cook or Manual on High pressure for 20 minutes with the Keep Warm setting off and the valve closed. • Use the quick-release method to bring the pot's pressure back to normal. Unlatch the lid and open the cooker. Use silicone cooking mitts or thick hot pads to remove the rack or steamer, letting the meat fall down into the liquid below. Use the edge of a large, metal spoon and a meat fork to break the meat up into little chunks, about the size of very small meatballs. Stir in the frozen vegetables. • Press the SAUTÉ button. Set it for HIGH, MORE or CUSTOM 400°F. Set the time for 5 Minutes and if necessary press START • Whisk the cream and flour in a small bowl until smooth. Once the liquid is simmering in the pot, add this cream mixture and whisk until bubbling. Turn off the SAUTÉ function. • To make the biscuit topping, stir the flour, baking powder, and salt in a medium bowl until uniform. Add the milk, melted butter or oil, and the egg. Continue stirring until the mixture has no dry ingredients in the bottom of the bowl. • Drop the mixture by eight blobs on top of the hot stew. Sprinkle the cheese (if using) over each of the blobs, then sprinkle each with a little paprika. Latch the lid onto the pot but do not engage the pressure valve. • Set the Instant Pot for SLOW COOK, set the level for HIGH and the valve must be OPEN. Set the timer for 30 minutes with the KEEP WARM setting off, and if necessary press the START button. • When the machine has finished cooking, turn it off and open the lid. Cool for a few minutes, then use a large cooking spoon to scoop the biscuits and stew into serving bowls.

Cheeseburger Pie

Ingredients for 6 servings:

1 lb ground beef preferably 93% lean ½ cup finely diced onion 1 tsp kosher salt 1 cup finely chopped spinach optional 1 cup shredded Cheddar cheese ½ cup baking mix 1 cup milk 2 eggs 1 cup Water Additional shredded cheddar for garnish optional

Directions and total time – 30-60 m

• Add ground beef and onion to the Instant Pot. Using the display panel select the SAUTE function. • Brown the meat until no pink remains. Drain and discard liquids. • Spread beef in the bottom of an IP-friendly casserole dish, sprinkle with salt, then layer spinach (if using) and shredded cheese. • In a medium bowl, whisk together baking mix, milk and eggs to form a thin batter. Pour evenly over the meat and cheese. Cover loosely with foil--do not seal. • Rinse out the pot, then pour in one cup of water and insert the steam rack. Carefully lower the casserole on to the steam rack. • Turn the pot off by selecting CANCEL, then secure the lid, making sure the vent is closed. • Using the display panel select the MANUAL or PRESSURE COOK function. Use the +/- keys and program the Instant Pot for 20 minutes. • When the time is up, let the pressure naturally release for 5 minutes, then quick-release the remaining pressure. • (Optional) Sprinkle additional shredded cheddar and set under the broiler for 3 - 5 minutes until cheese is bubbly. • Allow the casserole to set up for 5 - 10 minutes for easier serving.

Butternut Squash

Ingredients for 6 servings:

1 2 ½ pound butternut squash, cut into 1-inch cubes (about 6 cups) 1 cup water 1 teaspoon kosher salt

Directions and total time – 15-30 m

• Wash the outside of the squash well and trim the peel from the outside. Scoop out the seeds and cut into 1 inch cubes. • Place the cubes into the insert of a 6-quart Instant Pot with 1 cup of water. Set the Instant Pot pressure to HIGH and set time for 3 minutes if you want your squash to hold it's shape, or 4 minutes to make it even softer easier to mash. • When time is up, quick release and carefully remove the lid. Transfer the squash to a bowl, season with kosher salt and mash with a fork or a potato masher and season with butter or other flavorings if you like. Or, keep cubed and use in other recipes as suggested above.

Pulled Pork Carnitas

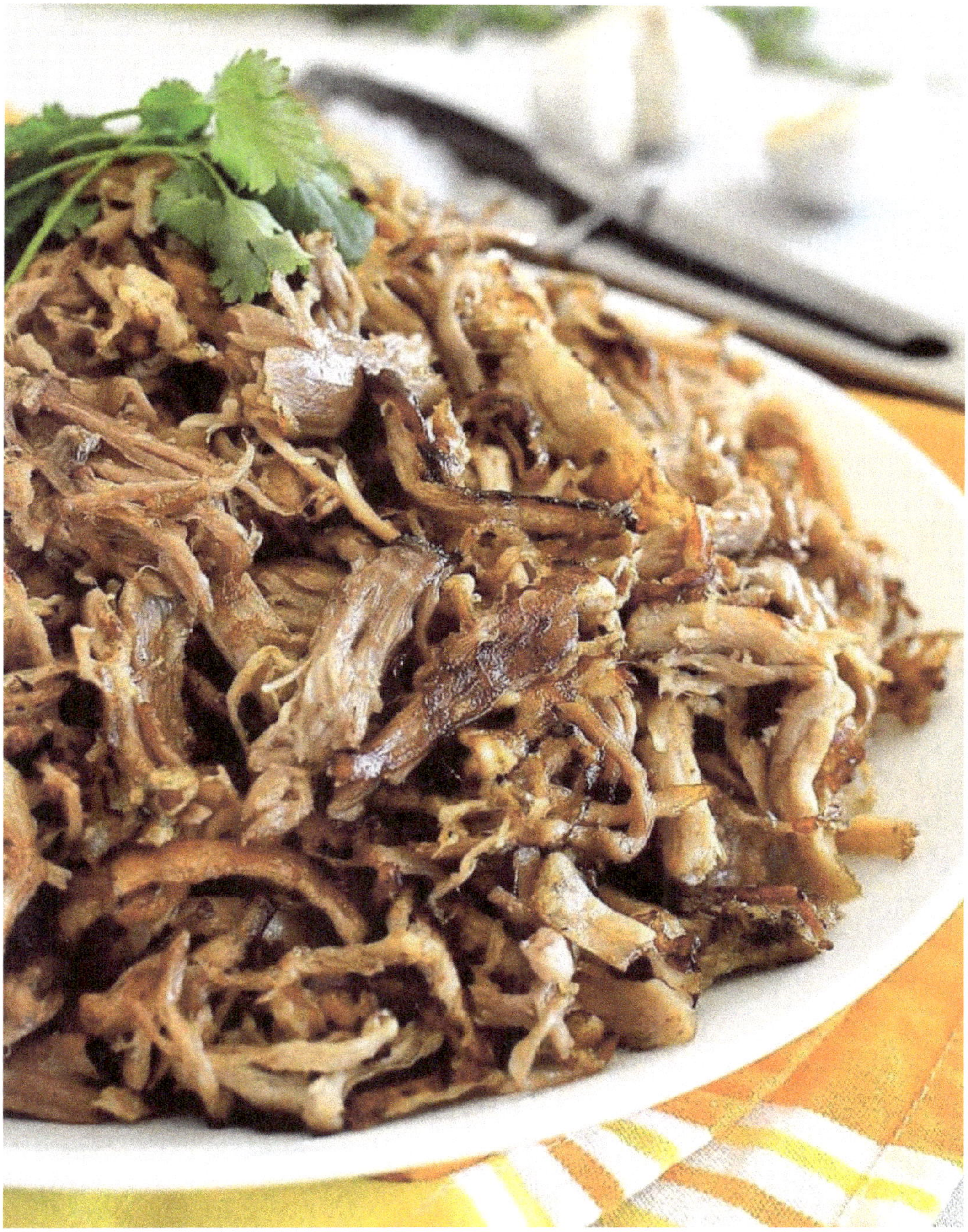

Ingredients for 8 servings:

For the spice rub: 4 tablespoons chili powder 1 tablespoon kosher salt (if using regular table salt, only use 2 teaspoons) 1 tablespoon brown sugar 2 teaspoons ground cumin 1 teaspoon cayenne 1 teaspoon dried oregano 1 teaspoon onion powder 1 teaspoon garlic powder ¼ teaspoon cinnamon Scant pinch of ground cloves For the pulled pork: 3 ½ pound boneless pork shoulder roast, cut into two pieces 2 tablespoons vegetable oil ¾ cup pineapple juice, orange juice, or water Optional toppings (pick a few!): Sliced avocado Sliced radishes Thinly sliced red or green cabbage Thinly sliced romaine lettuce Diced red onions Chopped tomatoes Crumbled cotija cheese Chopped cilantro Warm tortillas, corn or flour Fresh squeezed lime juice Salsa

Directions and total time – 1-2 h

• Season the pork: In a small bowl, combine the spice rub ingredients. Pat the pork dry with paper towels, then sprinkle with half of the spice rub. Turn and rub the spice into the pork until the pieces are evenly coated. • Let the pork sit 15 to 60 min: Leave the pork to absorb the rub and to take the chill off the meat, at least 15 minutes or up to an hour. (Room temperature pork will sear better). Sear the pork: Select the "Sauté" program on your pressure cooker and add the oil to the pot. (If you are using a stovetop pressure cooker, heat the oil over medium heat.) • Use a pair of tongs to lower the pork into the pot so the side with the most fat is facing down. Sear for 5 minutes. Flip it over and sear it for 5 more minutes. Both sides should be browned. • Sprinkle the remaining spice rub over the pork, then pour the pineapple juice over the top. • Pressure cook the pork: Place the lid on your pressure cooker. Make sure that the pressure regulator is set to the "Sealing" position. Select the "Manual" program on the pressure cooker and set the time to 1 hour and 15 minutes at high pressure. (For stovetop pressure cookers, cook for 60 minutes at high pressure.). It will take about 10 minutes for your pressure cooker to come up to pressure, and then the cooking time will begin. • Release the pressure: After the cooking time ends, let the pot sit and naturally release pressure for about 20 minutes, then vent the remaining steam. (For stovetop pressure cookers, perform a quick pressure release.) • Separate the pork and cooking liquid: Use tongs to transfer the pork to a large baking dish or sheet pan, but be very gentle -- the pork will be VERY tender and will fall apart easily. Then, use heat-proof mitts to lift the inner pot out of the pressure cooker, pour the cooking liquid into a fat separator, then pour the liquid back into the pot. Reserve the fat. (Alternatively, let the cooking liquid stand for about 10 minutes until the fat floats to the top, then use a shallow spoon to skim as much fat as possible from the surface.) • Reduce the cooking liquid: Return the pot to the pressure cooker, select the "Sauté" program, and let the cooking liquid reduce for 10 minutes. (If you are using a stovetop pressure cooker, do the same thing over medium heat.) • While the liquid is reducing, use a pair of forks to shred the pork. • Broil the pulled pork until crispy (optional for carnitas): To make crispy carnitas, place the pan of shredded pork 6 to 8 inches below the broiler and broil for 5 to 10 minutes until the tips and edges of the pork are browned and crispy. It's fine to skip this step if you're making a recipe where you don't need the pork to be crispy. • Toss the shredded pork with the reduced liquid and serve: Return the pork to the pot with the reduced cooking liquid and toss to coat the pork evenly. If the pork seems a little dry, add a tablespoon or two of the reserved fat. • Serve it in tacos with the fixings listed above, or in burritos or rice bowls, or on a tostada salad.

Keto Mac and Cheese

Ingredients for 4 servings:

4 tbsp grass-fed butter softened 1 cup full-fat Cheddar cheese shredded 1 cup full-fat Monterey Jack cheese shredded 1 head cauliflower chopped ½ cup heavy whipping cream ½ cup full-fat Parmesan cheese grated ½ tsp cayenne pepper ground ½ tsp freshly ground black pepper ½ tsp kosher salt

Directions and total time – 15 m

• Pour 2 cups of filtered water into the Instant Pot, then insert the trivet. In a large bowl, combine all ingredients, mixing thoroughly. Transfer this mixture into a well-greased, Instant Pot–friendly dish. • Place the dish onto the trivet, and cover loosely with aluminum foil. Close the lid, set the pressure release to Sealing, and select Manual/Pressure Cook. Set the Instant Pot to 5 minutes on high pressure, and let cook. • Once cooked, let the pressure naturally disperse from the Instant Pot for about 10 minutes, then carefully switch the pressure release to Venting. • Open the Instant Pot, and remove the dish. Let cool, serve, and enjoy!

Duck with Orange

Ingredients for 4 servings:

4 duck thigh quarters bone-in 1 tsp salt ½ tsp pepper 1 tbsp vegetable oil 1 cup chicken broth 1 cup orange juice ½ cup sugar zest from one orange 1 tbsp Grand Marnier (optional) 2 tbsp cornstarch mixed with 2 tablespoons water, for slurry thin orange slices for garnish

Directions and total time – 30-60 m • Trim any excess skin from the duck quarters. Sprinkle the meat, on all sides, with salt and pepper. • Press the Sauté button to heat the Instant Pot inner pot. When the display reads "Hot," add the 1 tablespoon of vegetable oil to coat the bottom. Place the duck pieces skin side down into the hot pot in a single layer. If the pieces are large, you may have to cook them in two batches. Sear each side of the meat until it is until golden brown, approximately 4 minutes per side. • Remove the duck from the pot in order to deglaze the pot. Add the chicken broth to the pot and scrape the bottom with a wooden spoon, making sure to scrape up all the brown bits. Add the orange juice and sugar to the pot, stirring constantly, until the sugar is dissolved, about 2 minutes. • Add the orange zest and stir the pot. Press Cancel to turn off the sauté function. • Place the duck pieces back into pot, skin side up. Secure the lid, ensuring the valve is turned to the Sealing position. Press the Pressure Cook button and set the time to 12 minutes. • When cooking is complete, let the pot sit for another 10 minutes, and then turn the valve to the Venting position to release any remaining pressure. Turn on the broiler while the pressure is releasing. • Remove the lid when all the pressure has released. Using tongs, transfer the duck pieces from the pot to a broiler pan. Place the pan under the broiler until the duck skin becomes crispy, after 5–10 minutes. • While the duck is under the broiler, press the Sauté button and add in the Grand Marnier (if using) and the cornstarch and water slurry, whisking the sauce constantly until it has thickened. Press Cancel to turn off the Sauté function. • Remove the duck from the oven, place it on a serving platter, and spoon the sauce over the top. Garnish the duck with thin slices of orange.

Chicken with Potato plus Rice

Ingredients for 8 servings: Marinade Ingredients: 1 tablespoon dark soy sauce 1 tablespoon light soy sauce ¼ teaspoon white pepper powder 2 tablespoon Water 1 tablespoon corn starch Other Ingredients: 2 tablespoons olive oil 1 green onion cut in 2-inch length pieces 1 piece Ginger fresh, sliced 1 star anise 3 cloves 400 grams chicken thighs. Boneless and skinless, cut to small pieces 2 cups chicken stock low sodium, or water 1 ½ tablespoons dark soy sauce 1 tablespoon light soy sauce ½ teaspoon salt 1 ⅓ cups white long rice 3 medium yellow potatoes peeled and cut in ¼ inch pieces 1 green onion finely chopped 1 tablespoon sesame oil

Directions and total time – 30-60 m • Mix the chicken meat and all marinade ingredients the night before. Store in a container with a lid and place in the fridge overnight. • Select Sauté, heat olive oil over medium-high heat. • Add in 1 green onion (cut in 2 inches), star anise, fresh ginger, cloves and cook for a minute. • Add the marinated chicken meat, stir frequently for about 3 to 4 minutes until outside of chicken turns light brown, set aside. • Transfer all cooked chicken with liquid into the Instant Pot. Add the chicken broth, dark and light soy sauces, salt, rice, and potatoes. • Close the lid, make sure the valve is set to "Sealing" position. Select the "Rice" function and allow to cook for 12 minutes by adjusting the time. • When time is done, wait for another 10 minutes then quick release the pressure and open the lid. • Stir in finely chopped green onion and sesame oil. Cover the pot with the lid and let the rice sit for 5 minutes before serving.

Tyrolese Egg Salad
(Ready in about 30 minutes | Servings 4)
Per serving: 342 Calories; 29.2g Fat; 7.2g Carbs; 12.7g Protein; 3.6g Sugars

Ingredients 6 eggs 1/2 pound green beans, trimmed 1 cup of water 3 slices prosciutto, chopped 1/2 cup green onions, chopped 1 carrot, shredded 1/2 cup mayonnaise 1 tablespoon apple cider vinegar 1 teaspoon yellow mustard 4 tablespoons Gorgonzola cheese, crumbled

Directions Pour the water into the Instant Pot; add a steamer basket to the bottom. Arrange the eggs in a steamer basket. Secure the lid. Choose "Manual" mode and High pressure; cook for 5 minutes. Once cooking is complete, use a natural pressure release; carefully remove the lid. Allow the eggs to cool for 15 minutes. Peel the eggs and cut them into slices. Then, add green beans and 1 cup of water to your Instant Pot. Secure the lid. Choose "Manual" mode and Low pressure; cook for 5 minutes. Once cooking is complete, use a quick pressure release; carefully remove the lid. Transfer green beans to a salad bowl. Add prosciutto, green onions, carrot, mayonnaise, vinegar, and mustard. Top with Gorgonzola cheese and sliced eggs. Enjoy!

Asian-Style Savory Egg Custard
(Ready in about 15 minutes | Servings 3)
Per serving: 234 Calories; 16.8g Fat; 3.6g Carbs; 16.4g Protein; 1.8g Sugars

Ingredients

3 eggs, well beaten 1 cup broth, preferably homemade Kosher salt and white pepper, to taste 1 tablespoon tamari sauce 1/2 tablespoon oyster sauce 1/2 cup Comté cheese, grated

Directions

Place the beaten eggs in a mixing bowl. Slowly and gradually, add broth, whisking constantly as you go. Season with salt and paper. Then, pour this mixture through a strainer. Add tamari sauce and oyster sauce. Pour the mixture into three ramekins. Now, cover the ramekins with a piece of foil. Place the ramekins on the metal trivet. Secure the lid. Choose "Manual" mode and Low pressure; cook for 7 minutes. Once cooking is complete, use a natural pressure release; carefully remove the lid. Top with cheese and serve immediately. Bon appétit!

Fluffy Scrambled Eggs

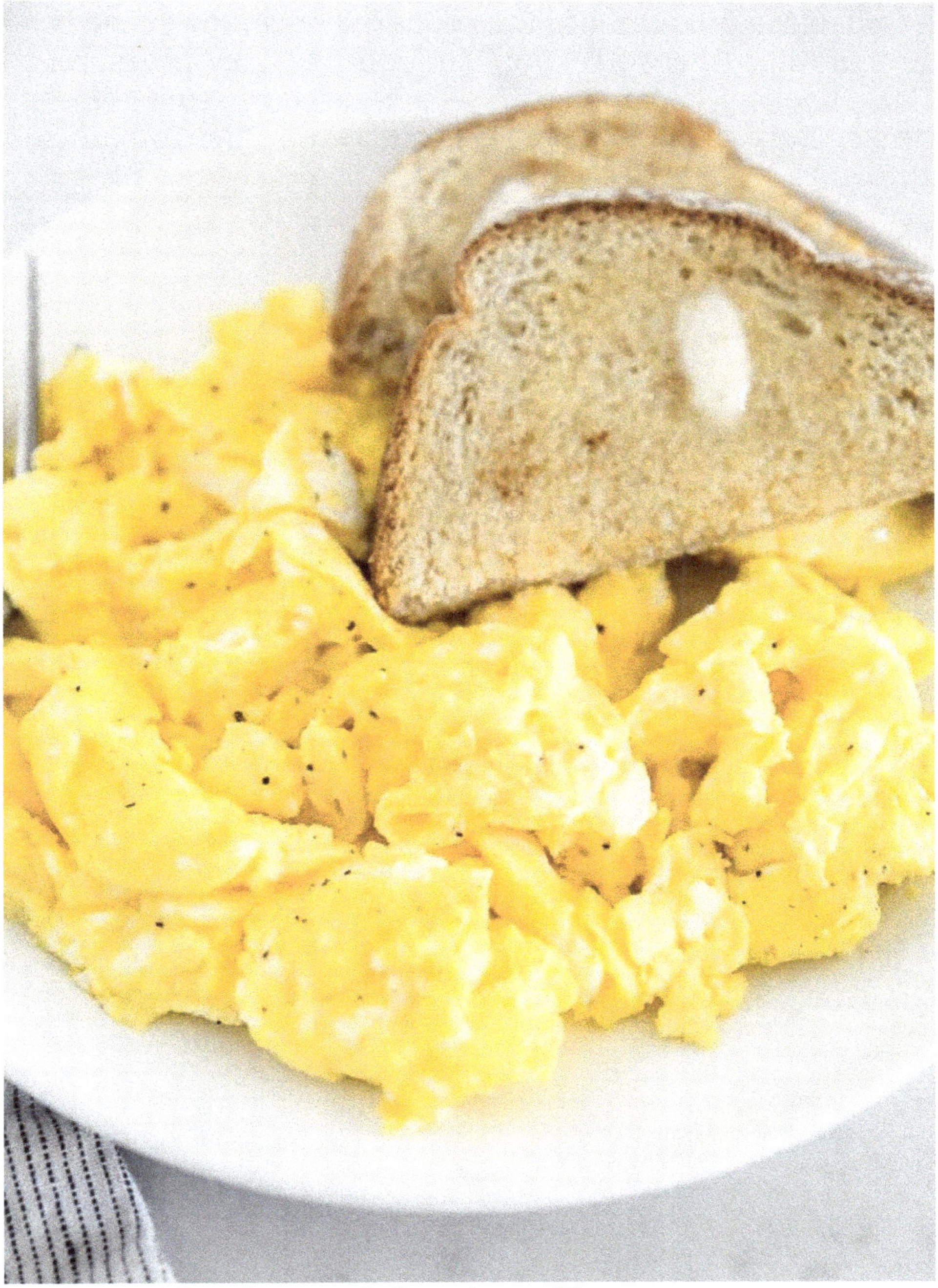

(Ready in about 10 minutes | Servings 2)

Per serving: 322 Calories; 25.6g Fat; 3.1g Carbs; 18.4g Protein; 1.3g Sugars

Ingredients

4 eggs, beaten 2 tablespoons full cream milk 1 tablespoon ghee, melted Salt, to taste 1/4 teaspoon ground black pepper, or more to taste 1/2 teaspoon smoked paprika

Directions

Begin by adding 1 cup of water and a metal rack to the Instant Pot. Spritz a heatproof bowl with a nonstick cooking spray. Mix all ingredients until well combined. Spoon the mixture into the prepared bowl; lower the bowl onto the rack. Secure the lid. Choose "Manual" mode and Low pressure; cook for 6 minutes. Once cooking is complete, use a natural pressure release; carefully remove the lid. Serve with a dollop of sour cream and tomatoes if desired. Bon appétit!

Broccoli with Asiago Cheese
(Ready in about 12 minutes | Servings 4)
Per serving: 160 Calories; 11.7g Fat; 5.3g Carbs; 10.1g Protein; 0.9g Sugars
Ingredients
1 tablespoon olive oil 2 tablespoons green onion, chopped 4 cloves garlic, pressed 1 pound broccoli, broken into florets 1 cup water 2 chicken bouillon cubes Sea salt and ground black pepper, to taste 3/4 cup Asiago cheese, shredded
Directions
Press the "Sauté" button to heat up your Instant Pot. Now, heat the oil and sweat green onions for 2 minutes. Stir in the garlic and continue to sauté an additional 30 seconds. Add broccoli, water, bouillon cubes, salt, and black pepper. Secure the lid. Choose "Manual" mode and High pressure; cook for 7 minutes. Once cooking is complete, use a natural pressure release; carefully remove the lid. Top with shredded cheese and serve immediately. Bon appétit!

Scamorza Open Tart

(Ready in about 30 minutes | Servings 4)

Per serving: 350 Calories; 25.1g Fat; 4.8g Carbs; 25.9g Protein; 2.9g Sugars

Ingredients

5 eggs, beaten 1/3 cup double cream Salt and ground black pepper, to taste 1 teaspoon cayenne pepper 5 ounces speck, chopped 1/4 cup scallions, chopped 1/2 cup Scamorza cheese, crumbled 1 bunch of Rucola, to serve

Directions

Begin by adding 1 cup of water and a metal rack to your Instant Pot. Then, spritz a heatproof bowl and set aside. In a mixing dish, thoroughly combine the eggs, cream, salt, black pepper, and cayenne pepper. Add chopped speck, scallions, and cheese. Spoon the mixture into the prepared heatproof bowl; cover with a piece of aluminum foil, making a foil sling. Secure the lid. Choose "Manual" mode and High pressure; cook for 25 minutes. Once cooking is complete, use a quick pressure release; carefully remove the lid. Garnish with Rucola and serve. Bon appétit!

Savory Muffins with Canadian Bacon
(Ready in about 10 minutes | Servings 4)
Per serving: 301 Calories; 41.3g Fat; 7.8g Carbs; 25.5g Protein; 3.5g Sugars

Ingredients

5 ounces Canadian bacon, sliced 1/2 cup Asiago cheese, shredded 4 eggs, beaten 2 tablespoons butter 2 tablespoons double cream Salt and black pepper, to taste 1/2 teaspoon red pepper flakes, crushed 1/2 teaspoon granulated garlic 1/4 cup shallots, minced 2 tablespoons coriander, chopped

Directions

Line muffin cups with bacon slices. Then, add a layer of cheese. In a mixing dish, whisk the eggs, butter, double cream, salt, black pepper, red pepper, and garlic. Pour the egg mixture over cheese. Sprinkle with minced shallots and coriander. Add 1 cup of water and a metal trivet to the Instant Pot. Now, place the muffin cups on the trivet. Secure the lid. Choose "Manual" mode and High pressure; cook for 6 minutes. Once cooking is complete, use a natural pressure release; carefully remove the lid. Allow the muffins to stand for a few minutes before removing from the cups. Bon appétit!

Peppery and Cheesy Deviled Eggs
(Ready in about 25 minutes | Servings 4)
Per serving: 264 Calories; 21.1g Fat; 6g Carbs; 11.7g Protein; 3.8g Sugars

Ingredients

6 eggs 1 teaspoon canola oil 1 onion, chopped 2 bell peppers, drained and chopped Seasoned salt and freshly ground black pepper, to taste 1/4 cup mayonnaise 1 teaspoon mustard 1 tablespoon fresh lemon juice 4 tablespoons Colby cheese, grated 1 teaspoon smoked Hungarian paprika

Directions

Pour the water into the Instant Pot; add a steamer basket to the bottom. Arrange the eggs in a steamer basket if you have one. Secure the lid. Choose "Manual" mode and High pressure; cook for 5 minutes. Once cooking is complete, use a natural pressure release; carefully remove the lid. Allow the eggs to cool for 15 minutes. Peel the eggs and separate egg whites from yolks. Press the "Sauté" button to heat up your Instant Pot; heat the oil. Now, sauté the onion along with peppers until softened. Season with salt and pepper. Add the reserved egg yolks to the pepper mixture. Stir in mayo, mustard, and lemon juice. Now, stuff the egg whites with this mixture. Top with grated Colby cheese and arrange the stuffed eggs on a serving platter. Afterwards, sprinkle Hungarian paprika over eggs and serve.

Three-Cheese and Beer Dip
(Ready in about 10 minutes | Servings 10)
Per serving: 220 Calories; 14.9g Fat; 2.9g Carbs; 18.1g Protein; 1.7g Sugars
Ingredients
16 ounces Cottage cheese, softened 5 ounces goat cheese, softened 1/2 teaspoon garlic powder 1 teaspoon stone-ground mustard 1/2 cup chicken stock, preferably homemade 1/2 cup lager beer 6 ounces pancetta, chopped 1 cup Monterey-Jack cheese, shredded 2 tablespoons fresh chives, roughly chopped
Directions
Add Cottage cheese, goat cheese, garlic powder, mustard, chicken stock, beer, and pancetta to the Instant Pot. Secure the lid. Choose "Manual" mode and High pressure; cook for 4 minutes. Once cooking is complete, use a quick pressure release; carefully remove the lid. Press the "Sauté" button to heat up your Instant Pot. Add Monterey-Jack cheese and stir until everything is thoroughly warmed. Sprinkle with fresh chopped chives and serve. Bon appétit!

Indian Egg Muffins

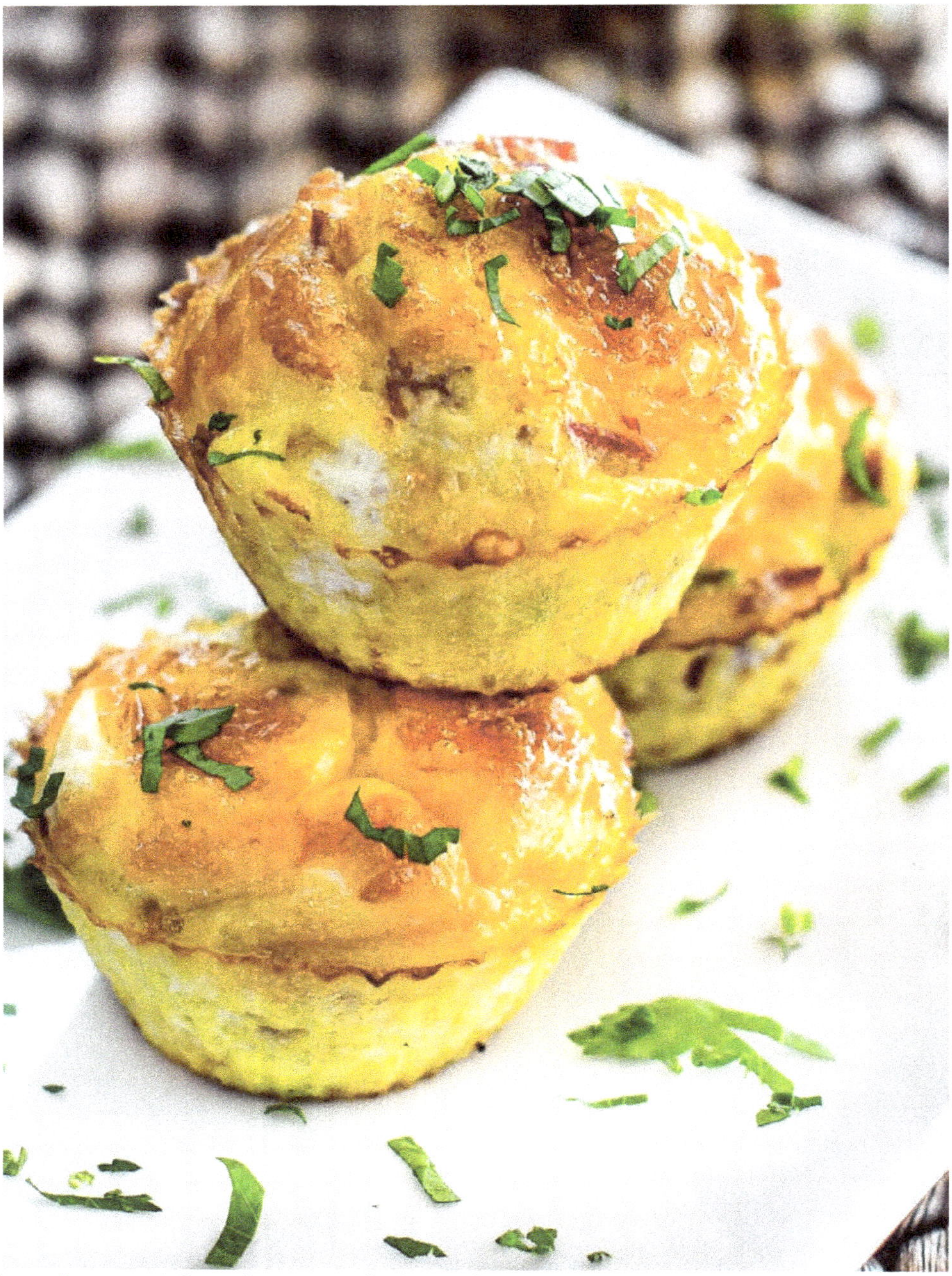

(Ready in about 10 minutes | Servings 5)
Per serving: 202 Calories; 13.7g Fat; 4.7g Carbs; 15.4g Protein; 2.6g Sugars

Ingredients

5 eggs Seasoned salt and ground black pepper, to taste 2 green chilies, minced 5 tablespoons feta cheese, crumbled 1/2 tablespoon Chaat masala powder 1 tablespoon fresh cilantro, finely chopped

Directions

Begin by adding 1 cup of water and a steamer basket to your Instant Pot. Mix all ingredients together; then, spoon the egg/cheese mixture into silicone muffin cups. Next, lower your muffin cups onto the steamer basket. Secure the lid. Choose "Manual" mode and High pressure; cook for 7 minutes. Once cooking is complete, use a quick pressure release; carefully remove the lid. Let your muffins sit for a few minutes before removing from the cups; serve warm. Bon appétit!

Manchego, Sausage and Vegetable Bake
(Ready in about 25 minutes | Servings 4)
Per serving: 344 Calories; 27.4g Fat; 3g Carbs; 20.3g Protein; 1.3g Sugars
Ingredients
8 slices pork sausage, chopped 1 ½ cups mushrooms, sliced 1 garlic clove, minced 1 cup kale leaves, torn into pieces 7 eggs 1/3 cup milk 1 cup Manchego cheese, shredded Sea salt and freshly ground black pepper, to taste
Directions
Press the "Sauté" button to heat up the Instant Pot. Now, cook the sausage until no longer pink. Then, add mushrooms and garlic; continue to cook until they are fragrant; turn off the Instant Pot; add kale and let it sit for 5 minutes. Wipe down your Instant Pot with a damp cloth. Add 1 cup of water and a metal rack. Spritz a baking dish that fits into your Instant Pot. In a mixing bowl, thoroughly combine the eggs, milk, cheese, salt and black pepper; add the sausage/vegetable mixture to the mixing bowl. Spoon the mixture into the baking dish. Lower the baking dish onto the rack. Secure the lid. Choose "Manual" mode and High pressure; cook for 15 minutes. Once cooking is complete, use a quick pressure release; carefully remove the lid. Enjoy!

Ooey Gooey, Cheesy Pizza
(Ready in about 20 minutes | Servings 6)
Per serving: 334 Calories; 25.1g Fat; 5.9g Carbs; 20.5g Protein; 2.8g Sugars
Ingredients
1 tablespoon olive oil 1 large-sized tomato, chopped 6 ounces pepperoni 1 yellow onion, chopped 2 bell peppers, chopped 1 cup mozzarella cheese, sliced 1/2 cup provolone cheese, sliced 3 eggs, whisked 1/2 teaspoon dried basil 1/2 teaspoon dried oregano 1/2 teaspoon dried rosemary 1/2 cup Kalamata olives, pitted and halved
Directions
Grease the bottom and sides of your Instant Pot with olive oil. Place 1/2 of chopped tomato on the bottom. Then, layer 3 ounces of pepperoni, 1/2 of yellow onion, 1 bell pepper, 1/2 cup of mozzarella cheese and 1/4 cup of provolone cheese. Continue layering until you run out of ingredients. Pour in the whisked eggs. Afterwards, sprinkle seasonings and olives over the top. Secure the lid. Choose "Manual" mode and High pressure; cook for 15 minutes. Once cooking is complete, use a natural pressure release; carefully remove the lid. Serve warm.

Egg Salad with Poppy Seed Dressing
(Ready in about 25 minutes | Servings 4)
Per serving: 340 Calories; 27.5g Fat; 8.1g Carbs; 16.4g Protein; 2.9g Sugars

Ingredients

5 medium-sized eggs 1/2 pound kale leaves, torn into pieces 1/2 cup radishes, sliced 1 white onion, thinly sliced 2 tablespoons champagne vinegar 1/2 tablespoon poppy seeds Sea salt and white pepper, to taste 1/2 teaspoon cayenne pepper 1 teaspoon yellow mustard 1/4 cup extra-virgin olive oil 3 ounces goat cheese, crumbled

Directions

Pour 1 cup of water into the Instant Pot; add a steamer basket to the bottom. Arrange the eggs in the steamer basket. Secure the lid. Choose "Manual" mode and High pressure; cook for 5 minutes. Once cooking is complete, use a natural pressure release; carefully remove the lid. Allow the eggs to cool for 15 minutes. Then, place them in your refrigerator and reserve. Then, place kale in the steamer basket. Secure the lid. Choose "Manual" mode and High pressure; cook for 1 minute. Once cooking is complete, use a quick pressure release; carefully remove the lid. Now, place radishes and onion in a salad bowl. Add kale and sliced eggs. In a mixing dish, thoroughly combine vinegar, poppy seeds, salt, white pepper, cayenne pepper, and olive oil. Pour the dressing over your salad. Top with goat cheese and serve well-chilled. Bon appétit!

Egg Curry in a Hurry

(Ready in about 20 minutes | Servings 6)

Per serving: 253 Calories; 19.7g Fat; 4.9g Carbs; 13.9g Protein; 2.5g Sugars

Ingredients

1 ½ tablespoons butter, melted 1 yellow onion, chopped 1 ½ tablespoons curry paste 2 ripe tomatoes, peeled and chopped 1 cup water 7 eggs, whisked 1/2 cup cheddar cheese, grated

Directions

Press the "Sauté" button to heat up the Instant Pot. Now, warm the butter; once hot, sauté the onion until softened and fragrant. Add the remaining ingredients and stir to combine. Secure the lid. Choose "Manual" mode and High pressure; cook for 10 minutes. Once cooking is complete, use a quick pressure release; carefully remove the lid. Enjoy!

Egg Drop Soup with Gorgonzola
(Ready in about 20 minutes | Servings 4
Per serving: 163 Calories; 11.7g Fat; 3.1g Carbs; 10.8g Protein; 1.1g Sugars

Ingredients

1 tablespoon olive oil 1 carrot, chopped 1 clove garlic, minced 3 cups beef bone broth 1/2 cup water 2 eggs, slightly whisked Sea salt and ground black pepper, to your liking 1 teaspoon celery seeds 1/2 teaspoon paprika 1/2 cup Gorgonzola cheese, crumbled 1 heaping tablespoon fresh chives, minced

Directions

Press the "Sauté" button to heat up the Instant Pot. Now, heat the olive oil and cook the carrot and garlic until fragrant. Add broth and water. Secure the lid. Choose "Manual" mode and High pressure; cook for 10 minutes. Once cooking is complete, use a quick pressure release; carefully remove the lid. Then, mix the eggs, salt, black pepper, celery seeds, paprika, and cheese until well blended. Stir this mixture into the Instant Pot and press the "Sauté" button. Whisk until heated through. Serve in individual bowls, garnished with fresh chives. Enjoy!

Kid-Friendly Mini Frittatas

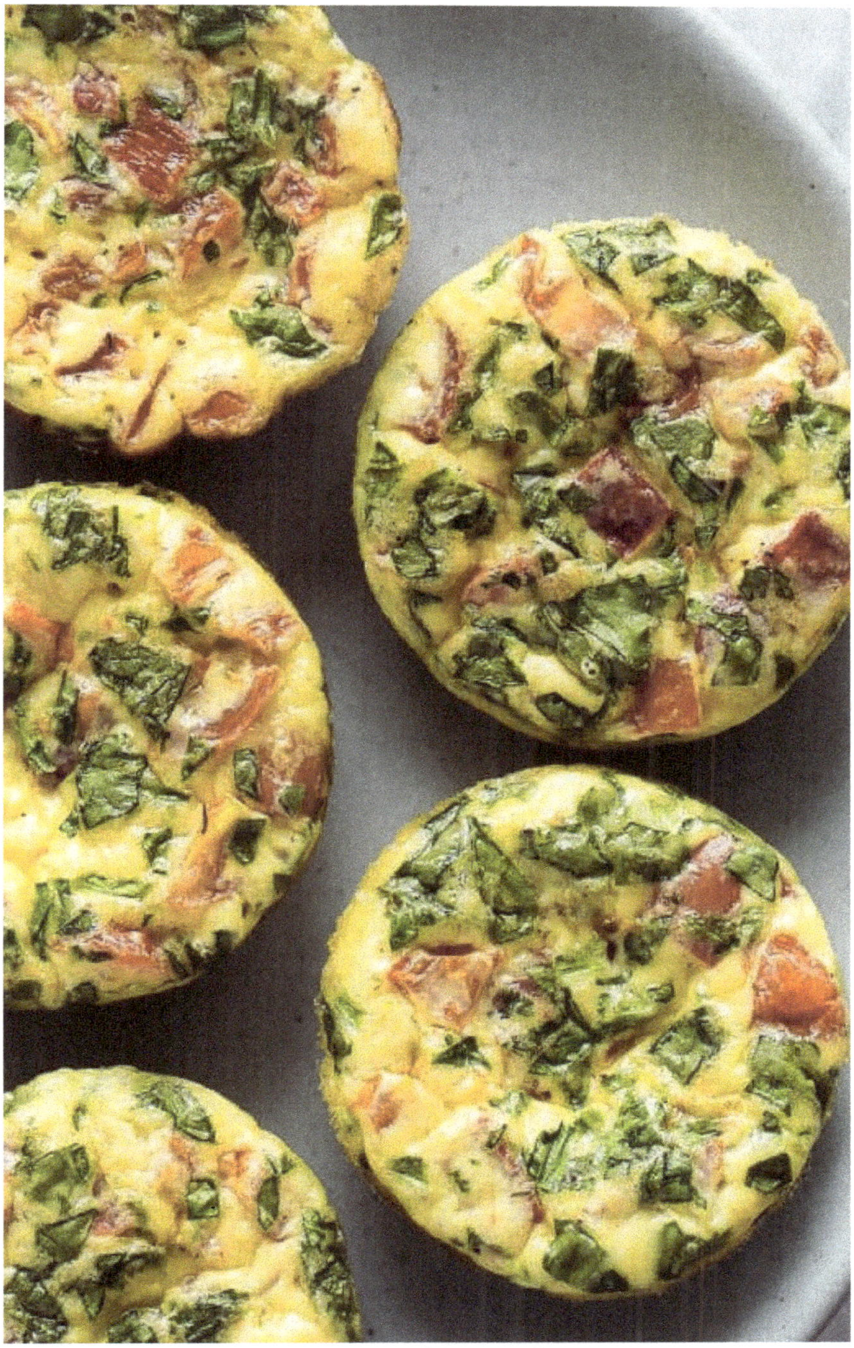

(Ready in about 15 minutes | Servings 4)

Per serving: 314 Calories; 25.6g Fat; 2.9g Carbs; 16.7g Protein; 1.7g Sugars

Ingredients

4 eggs 1/4 cup full-fat milk Sea salt, to taste 1/4 teaspoon ground black pepper 1/4 teaspoon cayenne pepper, or more to taste 1/2 teaspoon granulated garlic 1/3 teaspoon ground bay leaf 1/2 teaspoon dried dill weed 1 cup Chorizo sausage, chopped 1/2 cup green onions, chopped

Directions

Prepare your Instant Pot by adding 1 cup of water and a metal trivet to the bottom of the inner pot. Thoroughly combine all ingredients until everything is well mixed. Spoon the mixture into silicone molds. Lower the silicone molds onto the trivet. Secure the lid. Choose "Manual" mode and High pressure; cook for 7 minutes. Once cooking is complete, use a quick pressure release; carefully remove the lid. Bon appétit!

Asparagus and Colby Cheese Frittatas
(Ready in about 25 minutes | Servings 6
Per serving: 272 Calories; 21.1g Fat; 4.7g Carbs; 15.5g Protein; 2.3g Sugars
Ingredients
1 tablespoon butter, softened 1/2 cup leeks, chopped 2 garlic cloves, minced 10 asparagus spears, chopped 6 eggs, beaten 4 tablespoons milk 3 tablespoons cream cheese Kosher salt and white pepper, to taste 1/2 teaspoon thyme, minced 1/2 teaspoon rosemary, minced 1 cup Colby cheese, shredded
Directions
Press the "Sauté" button to heat up the Instant Pot. Now, melt the butter and sauté the leeks until softened. Add garlic and cook an additional 30 seconds. Turn off your Instant Pot. Add the remaining ingredients and mix to combine. Spoon the mixture into lightly greased ramekins. Wipe down your Instant Pot with a damp cloth. Place 1 cup of water and a rack in your Instant Pot. Lower the ramekins onto the rack. Cover them with a piece of foil. Secure the lid. Choose "Soup/Broth" mode and Low pressure; cook for 20 minutes. Once cooking is complete, use a quick pressure release; carefully remove the lid. Bon appétit!

Two-Cheese and Mustard Green Dip
(Ready in about 10 minutes | Servings 8)
Per serving: 49 Calories; 3.1g Fat; 1.4g Carbs; 3.9g Protein; 0.8g Sugars

Ingredients

1 cup mustard greens, chopped 4 ounces Cottage cheese, at room temperature 1/2 cup goat cheese, at room temperature Salt and ground black pepper, to taste 1 teaspoon Dijon mustard

Directions

Simply throw all of the above ingredients into your Instant Pot. Secure the lid. Choose "Manual" mode and Low pressure; cook for 3 minutes. Once cooking is complete, use a quick pressure release; carefully remove the lid. Serve warm and enjoy!

Portobello Mushrooms Baked Eggs and Cheese
(Ready in about 10 minutes | Servings 4)
Per serving: 256 Calories; 18.6g Fat; 5.3g Carbs; 17g Protein; 2.9g Sugars
Ingredients
4 medium-sized Portobello mushrooms, stems removed 4 eggs 1 red bell pepper, deveined and chopped 1 green bell pepper, deveined and chopped Sea salt and ground black pepper, to your liking 1/2 teaspoon cayenne pepper 1/2 teaspoon dried dill weed 1 cup Pepper-Jack cheese, grated
Directions
Start by adding 1 cup of water and a metal trivet to your Instant Pot. Spritz Portobello mushrooms with a nonstick cooking spray. Mix the eggs, pepper, salt, black pepper, cayenne pepper, and dill; mix until everything is well combined. Spoon this mixture into the prepared mushrooms caps. Place the stuffed mushrooms onto the metal trivet. Secure the lid. Choose "Manual" mode and High pressure; cook for 6 minutes. Once cooking is complete, use a quick pressure release; carefully remove the lid. Top with shredded cheese. Bon appétit!

Eggs with Peppers in Tomato Sauce
(Ready in about 10 minutes | Servings 4)
Per serving: 171 Calories; 12.2g Fat; 7.6g Carbs; 8.4g Protein; 4.1g Sugars

Ingredients

2 tablespoons olive oil 1 shallot, diced 1 teaspoon garlic paste 2 bell peppers, diced Salt and freshly ground black pepper, to taste 1 teaspoon cayenne pepper 1 teaspoon dried basil 2 ripe tomatoes, puréed 5 eggs 2 heaping tablespoons chives, chopped

Directions

Press the "Sauté" button to heat up your Instant Pot. Now, heat the olive oil and sauté the shallot until tender and aromatic. Add the garlic paste, peppers, salt, black pepper, cayenne pepper, basil, and tomatoes. Then, crack the eggs into the vegetable mixture. Secure the lid. Choose "Manual" mode and Low pressure; cook for 5 minutes. Once cooking is complete, use a quick pressure release; carefully remove the lid. Serve garnished with chopped chives. Enjoy!

Mélange with Spanish Chorizo
(Ready in about 25 minutes | Servings 6)
Per serving: 385 Calories; 30.2g Fat; 6.5g Carbs; 21.2g Protein; 3.1g Sugars
Ingredients
8 eggs 2 tablespoons olive oil 1/2 cup leeks, chopped 1 carrot, chopped 1 teaspoon fresh garlic, minced 1/2 cup Spanish chorizo, finely diced 2 ripe Roma tomatoes, puréed 2 sprigs fresh thyme 2 sprigs fresh rosemary 1 bay leaf Sea salt and ground black pepper, to taste 1/2 teaspoon smoked paprika 1 cup chicken stock 1 cup white cheddar cheese, shredded
Directions
Place 1 cup of water and a steamer basket in your Instant Pot. Now, arrange the eggs on the steamer basket. Secure the lid. Choose "Manual" mode and Low pressure; cook for 5 minutes. Once cooking is complete, use a quick pressure release; carefully remove the lid. Allow the eggs to cool and then, chop them roughly. Press the "Sauté" button to heat up your Instant Pot. Now, heat the olive oil until sizzling. Once hot, cook the leeks until they are softened. Add the carrot, garlic and chorizo; cook an additional minute or until just softened. Add tomatoes, thyme, rosemary, bay leaf, salt, pepper, paprika, and stock. Add the reserved hard-boiled eggs. Secure the lid. Choose "Manual" mode and High pressure; cook for 10 minutes. Once cooking is complete, use a quick pressure release; carefully remove the lid. Top with cheddar cheese, cover with the lid and let it sit until the cheese is completely melted. Bon appétit!

Ground Meat and Cheese Dip

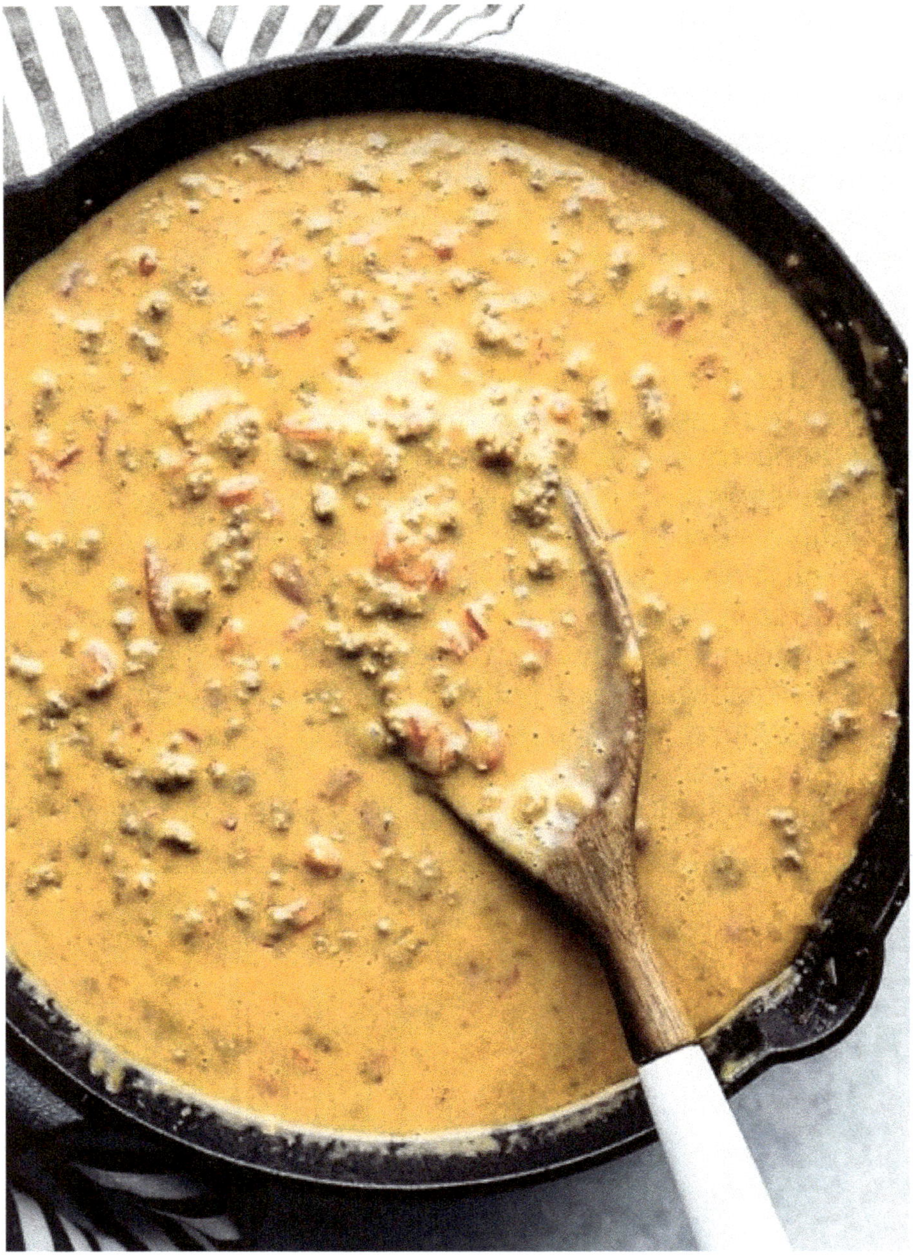

(Ready in about 10 minutes | Servings 10

Per serving: 254 Calories; 17.9g Fat; 3.9g Carbs; 18.8g Protein; 2.6g Sugars

Ingredients

2 teaspoons olive oil 1 yellow onion, chopped 1/2 pound ground pork 1/2 pound ground beef 1 teaspoon chili powder Sea salt, to taste 1/3 teaspoon freshly ground black pepper 1 tomato, chopped 1/3 cup salsa verde 1/2 cup chicken stock 7 ounces Mascarpone cheese, room temperature 5 ounces Colby cheese, grated

Directions

Press the "Sauté" button to heat up your Instant Pot. Now, heat the oil and cook the onion until tender. Next, cook the pork and beef until no longer pink, about 4 minutes. After that, add chili powder, salt, black pepper, tomato, and salsa verde. Secure the lid. Choose "Manual" mode and High pressure; cook for 5 minutes. Once cooking is complete, use a natural pressure release; carefully remove the lid. Add cheese and cover with the lid. Let it sit in the residual heat until everything is well combined. Enjoy!

Bacon, Egg, Lettuce Tomato
(Ready in about 10 minutes | Servings 4)
Per serving: 258 Calories; 20.1g Fat; 5.5g Carbs; 14.1g Protein; 3.1g Sugars
Ingredients
4 eggs Salt and freshly ground black pepper, to taste 4 slices bacon 8 leaves lettuce 1 large-sized tomato, sliced
Directions
Add 1 cup of water and a metal trivet to the Instant Pot. Spritz four silicone cups with a nonstick cooking spray. Crack an egg into each cup. Then, lower the silicone cups onto the metal trivet. Secure the lid. Choose "Steam" mode and High pressure; cook for 4 minutes. Once cooking is complete, use a quick pressure release; carefully remove the lid. Season your eggs with salt and pepper. Press the "Sauté" button to heat up your Instant Pot. Once hot, cook the bacon until crisp and browned. Divide lettuce leaves between four serving plates. Add bacon slice on each serving; place a few slices of tomato on each serving. Top with poached eggs and serve warm. Bon appétit!

Green Beans with Cheese and Eggs
(Ready in about 10 minutes | Servings 4)
Per serving: 249 Calories; 19.4g Fat; 7.2g Carbs; 12.2g Protein; 2.6g Sugars

Ingredients

2 tablespoons olive oil 2 garlic cloves, pressed 1 pound green beans, sliced 4 eggs, slightly whisked Salt and freshly ground black pepper, to taste 1 cup stock, preferably homemade 1 cup feta cheese, crumbled

Directions

Press the "Sauté" button to heat up your Instant Pot. Now, heat the olive oil until sizzling. Once hot, stir in garlic and cook for 40 seconds or until fragrant. Add green beans, eggs, salt, pepper, and stock. Secure the lid. Choose "Manual" mode and Low pressure; cook for 3 minutes. Once cooking is complete, use a quick pressure release; carefully remove the lid. Afterwards, add feta cheese and serve immediately.

Indian Egg Bhurji
(Ready in about 15 minutes | Servings 4
Per serving: 259 Calories; 20.6g Fat; 4.6g Carbs; 13.4g Protein; 2.6g Sugars
Ingredients
1 ½ tablespoons sesame oil 1/2 yellow onion, chopped 2 garlic cloves, minced 1 (1/2-inch) piece fresh ginger, grated 2 cups Cremini mushrooms, sliced 4 eggs, beaten 4 tablespoons full-fat milk Table salt and ground black pepper, to taste 1/4 teaspoon turmeric 1 teaspoon garam masala 1/2 cup Pepper-Jack cheese, preferably freshly grated
Directions
Press the "Sauté" button to heat up your Instant Pot. Heat the oil and cook the onion until they are caramelized; add a splash of water if needed. After that, stir in the garlic, ginger, and mushrooms; continue to cook an additional 1 minute or until fragrant. Add beaten eggs, milk, salt, pepper, turmeric, and garam masala. Secure the lid. Choose "Manual" mode and High pressure; cook for 7 minutes. Once cooking is complete, use a quick pressure release; carefully remove the lid. Add Pepper-Jack cheese and put the lid on the Instant Pot. Let it sit in the residual heat for 3 to 5 minutes. Serve warm and enjoy!

Winter Bacon and Leek Quiche
(Ready in about 35 minutes | Servings 6)
Per serving: 231 Calories; 15.2g Fat; 6.9g Carbs; 16.5g Protein; 3.1g Sugars

Ingredients

4 slices Canadian bacon, chopped 1 cup leeks, chopped 1 garlic clove, minced 8 eggs 1/2 cup half-and-half 1/2 cup cream cheese, room temperature Seasoned salt and ground black pepper, to taste 1 tablespoon dried sage, crushed 1/2 teaspoon marjoram 1/2 cup Swiss cheese, freshly grated

Directions

Press the "Sauté" button to heat up your Instant Pot. Once hot, cook the bacon until crisp and browned. Add the leeks and garlic and cook 1 minute more. Add the eggs, half-and-half, cream cheese, salt, black pepper, sage and marjoram. Grease a baking pan with a nonstick cooking spray. Spoon the bacon/egg mixture into the prepared baking pan. Now, add 1 cup of water and a metal trivet to the Instant Pot; lower the baking pan onto the trivet. Secure the lid. Choose "Meat/Stew" mode and High pressure; cook for 25 minutes. Once cooking is complete, use a quick pressure release; carefully remove the lid. Add Swiss cheese and cover with the lid; let it sit in the residual heat for 5 minutes. Serve with Dijon mustard.

Honey Baked Ham

Ingredients for 6-8 servings:

Glaze: 4 garlic cloves minced 4 tbs orange marmalade/jam 4 tbs Dijon mustard 3 tbs brown sugar 1 orange zested 1 cup Freshly Squeezed Orange Juice 1 tbs fresh rosemary Ham: 2 lb fully cooked smoked ham

Directions and total time – 30-60 m

• In a small bowl mix the garlic, orange marmalade (or jam), Dijon mustard, brown sugar, orange zest and orange juice. Use a hand blender to blend all the ingredients until you get a smooth glaze. Add the fresh thyme to the mixture. • Set your Instant Poti oven on Bake function at 360°F for 50 minutes. Place the ham on top of the baking pan and pour the glaze over the ham. • The ham is done when it is heated (the internal temperature should be ~145°F), and the glaze develops a golden-brown color.

Italian-Style Braised Pork Chops

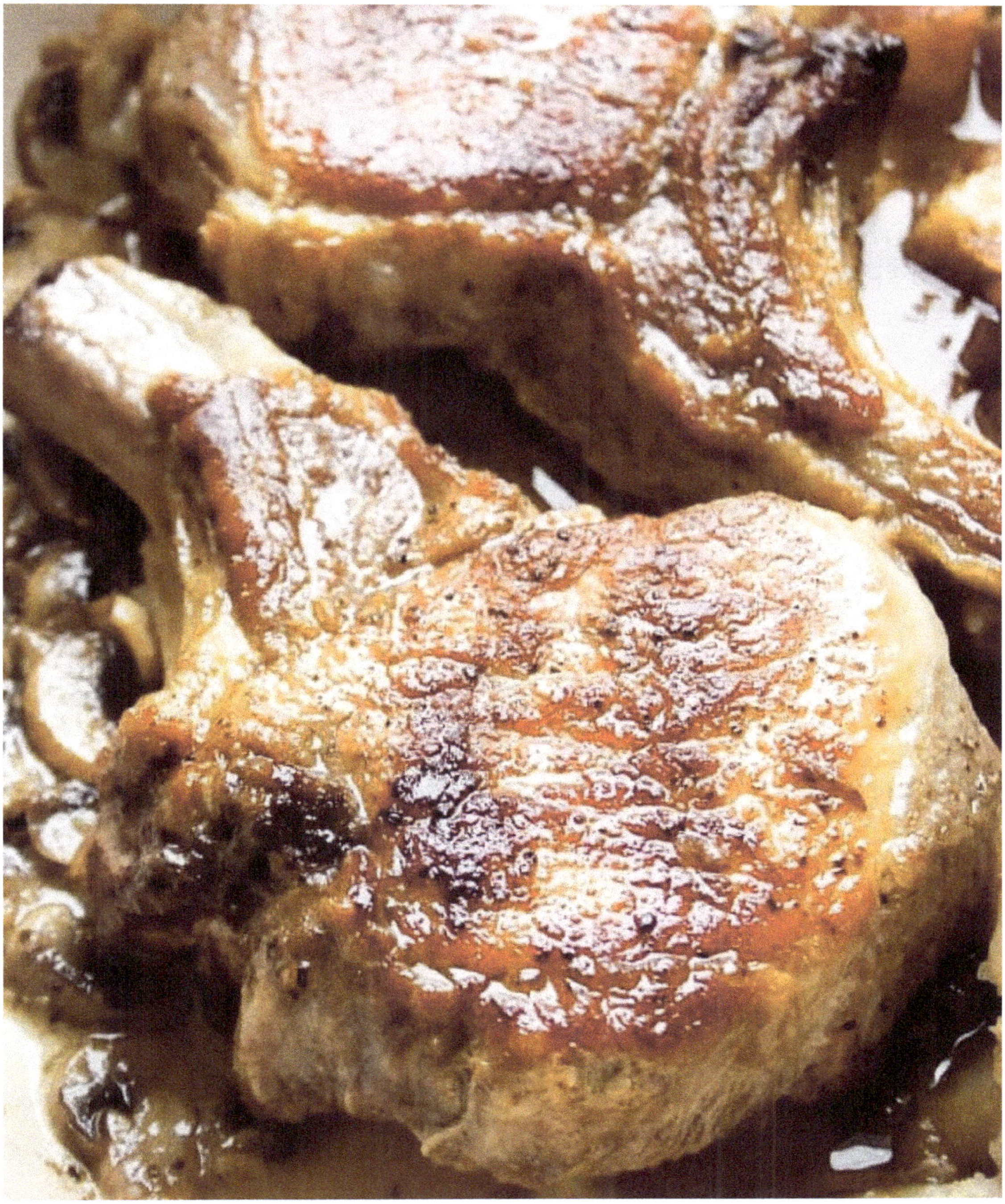

Ingredients for 4 servings:

1 cup chicken broth 2 tbsp balsamic vinegar 2 tsp stemmed thyme leaves or 1 tsp dried thyme ¼ tsp grated fresh nutmeg or ⅛ tsp ground nutmeg ¼ tsp red pepper flakes ¼ tsp table salt 4 cups frozen bell pepper strips 16-ounce bag 4 frozen center-cut boneless pork loin chops 6-8-ounce each

Directions and total time – 30 m

• Stir the broth, vinegar, thyme, nutmeg, red pepper flakes, and salt in an Instant Pot. Mix in the frozen pepper strips, then set the pork chops in the pot so they stand up on their sides and lean against each other and the side of the insert with room between each for liquid and pepper strips (in other words, not in a stack). Lock the lid onto the pot. • Option 1 Max Pressure Cooker • Press Pressure cook on Max pressure for 16 minutes with the Keep Warm setting off. • Optional 2 All Pressure Cookers • Press Meat/Stew, Pressure Cook or Manual on High pressure for 20 minutes with the Keep Warm setting off. The vent must be closed. • Use the quick-release method to bring the pot's pressure back to normal. Unlatch the lid and open the cooker. Transfer the pork chops to serving plates and spoon some of the sauce and peppers over each.

Spinach and Feta Stuffed Chicken
Ingredients for 4 servings:
4 boneless, skinless chicken breasts butterflied (6 ounce ½ cup frozen spinach ⅓ cup crumbled feta cheese 1 ¼ tsp salt divided ¼ tsp pepper ¼ tsp garlic powder ¼ tsp dried oregano ¼ tsp dried parsley 2 tbsp coconut oil 1 cup Water
Directions and total time – 20 m2
• Pound chicken breasts to ¼-inch thickness. In medium bowl, mix frozen spinach and feta and add ¼ teaspoon salt. Evenly divide mixture and spoon onto chicken breasts. • Close chicken breasts and secure with toothpicks or butcher's string. Sprinkle remaining seasonings onto chicken. Press the Sauté button and add coconut oil to Instant Pot. Sear each chicken breast until golden brown (this may take two batches). Press the Cancel button. • Remove chicken and set aside briefly. Pour water into Instant Pot and scrape bottom to remove any chicken or seasoning that is stuck on. Place steam rack into pot. • Place chicken on steam rack and click lid closed. Press 'Pressure Cook' and adjust time for 15 minutes. When timer beeps, allow a 15-minute natural release, then quick-release the remaining pressure. Serve warm with favorite white sauce if desired.

Pot Roast

Ingredients for 6 servings:

2 ½ lbs boneless beef chuck roast (up to 3 lbs 1 tbsp vegetable oil ½ cup dry red wine 2 large Onions cut into large chunks or wedges (about 3 cups) 5 large carrots peeled and cut into 2 inchpieces or2 ½ cups of baby cut carrots 1 lbs whole baby red potatoes or medium red potatoes cut in half 2 sprigs fresh thyme leaves 1 can Condensed Cream of Mushroom Soup 10 ½ ounces

Directions and total time – 1-2 h

• Cut the beef in half crosswise (for quicker cooking), then season with salt and pepper. On a 6 quart Instant Pot, select the Saute setting. Heat the oil. Add the beef (in batches, if needed) and cook for 15 minutes or until well browned on all sides. Remove the beef from the pot. Add the wine and cook, stirring to scrape up the browned bits from the bottom of the pot. Press Cancel. • Layer the onions, carrots, potatoes, thyme and beef in the Instant Pot. Spoon the soup over the beef (the order is important, so don't stir until after the cooking is done). • Lock the lid and close the pressure release valve. Pressure cook on High pressure, setting the timer to 45 minutes (timer will begin counting down once pressure is reachedit takes about 10 minutes). When done, press Cancel and use the quick release method to release the pressure. • Remove the beef to a serving plate, cover and keep warm. Select the Saute setting and cook the vegetables and gravy for 10 minutes or until the gravy is slightly thickened. Remove and discard the thyme. Season to taste. Slice the beef and serve with the vegetables and gravy.

Shrimp Gumbo

Ingredients for 6 servings:

¼ cup vegetable oil ¼ cup all-purpose flour 4 stalks celery chopped 1 large yellow onion peeled and diced 1 large green bell pepper seeded and diced 2 garlic cloves peeled and minced 1 can diced tomatoes 14.5 ounce ¼ tsp dried thyme ¼ tsp cayenne pepper 2 bay leaves 1 tbsp filé powder 2 tsp Worcestershire sauce 4 cups Seafood Stock 1 lb smoked sausage sliced 1 lb medium shrimp peeled and deveined ¼ tsp salt ¼ tsp ground black pepper 2 cups cooked long-grain rice

Directions and total time – 30-60 m

• Press the Sauté button on the Instant Pot and heat oil. Add flour and cook, stirring constantly, until flour is medium brown in color, about 15 minutes. • Add celery, onion, green pepper, garlic, and tomatoes and cook, stirring constantly, until the vegetables are tender, about 8 minutes. Add thyme, cayenne, bay leaves, filé, Worcestershire sauce, and stock and stir well, making sure nothing is stuck to the bottom of the pot, then add sausage. Press the Cancel button. • Close lid and set steam release to Sealing, then press the Manual button and adjust cook time to 8 minutes. When the timer beeps, quick release the pressure. Open lid and stir in shrimp, salt, and black pepper. Press the Cancel button, then press the Sauté button and cook for 8 minutes, or until shrimp are cooked through. Discard bay leaves. Serve hot over rice.

Beer Cheese Soup

Ingredients for 8 servings:

3 tbsp unsalted butter 2 medium carrots peeled and chopped 2 stalks celery chopped 1 medium onion peeled and chopped 1 clove garlic peeled and minced 1 tsp dried mustard ½ tsp smoked paprika ¼ cup all-purpose flour 1 bottle lager beer or ale 12-ounce 4 cups chicken broth ½ cup heavy cream 2 cups shredded sharp cheddar cheese 1 cup shredded smoked Gouda cheese

Directions and total time – 30-60 m

• Press the Sauté button on the Instant Pot and melt butter. Add carrots, celery, and onion. Cook, stirring often, until softened, about 5 minutes. Add garlic and cook until fragrant, about 30 seconds, then add mustard and paprika and stir well. • Add flour and stir well to combine, then cook for 1 minute. Slowly stir in beer, scraping the bottom of pot well, then add broth. Press the Cancel button. • Close lid, set steam release to Sealing, press the Manual button, and set time to 5 minutes. When the timer beeps, let pressure release naturally, about 15 minutes. Open lid and purée mixture with an immersion blender. Stir in cream, then stir in cheese 1 cup

Tahini Lamb Meatballs with Couscous and Pickled Onions
Ingredients for 4 servings:
Lamb Meatballs and Couscous Ingredients: ½ cup Tahini Sauce divided 3 tbsp panko bread crumbs 1 lb ground lamb ¼ cup chopped fresh mint divided 1 tsp ground cinnamon divided 1 tsp ground cumin divided ¾ tsp table salt divided 1 tbsp extra-virgin olive oil 1 onion chopped fine ⅛ tsp cayenne pepper 1 cup chicken broth plus extra as needed 1 cup couscous ½ cup jarred roasted red peppers rinsed, patted dry, and chopped 1 tbsp teaspoon grated lemon zest plus 1juice ⅓ cup Quick Pickled Onions Tahini Sauce Ingredients: ½ cup tahini ½ cup Water ¼ cup lemon juice (2 lemons) 2 garlic cloves minced Quick Pickled Onions Ingredients: 1 cup red wine vinegar ⅓ cup sugar ⅛ tsp table salt 1 red onion halved and sliced thin through root end
Directions and total time – 1-2 h Tahini Sauce Instructions • Whisk all Tahini sauce ingredients in bowl until smooth (mixture will appear broken at first). Season with salt and pepper to taste. Let sit at room temperature for at least 30 minutes to allow flavors to meld. (Sauce can be refrigerated for up to 4 days; bring to room temperature before serving.) Quick Pickled Onions Instructions • Microwave vinegar, sugar, and salt in medium bowl until simmering, 1 to 2 minutes. Add onion and let sit, stirring occasionally, for 45 minutes. Drain onion and return to now-empty bowl. (Drained onions can be refrigerated for up to 1 week.) Lamb Meatballs and Couscous • Using fork, mash ¼ cup Tahini Sauce and panko together in bowl to form paste. Add ground lamb, 2 tablespoons mint, ½ teaspoon cinnamon, ½ teaspoon cumin, and ½ teaspoon salt, and knead with hands until thoroughly combined. Pinch off and roll mixture into twelve 1 ½ inch meatballs. • Using highest Sauté function, heat oil in Instant Pot until shimmering. Add onion and remaining ¼ teaspoon salt and cook until onion is softened, about 5 minutes. Stir in remaining ½ teaspoon cinnamon, remaining ½ teaspoon cumin, and cayenne and cook until fragrant, about 30 seconds. Stir in broth, scraping up any browned bits. Add meatballs to pot. Lock lid in place and close pressure release valve. Select Pressure Cook function and cook for 1 minute. • Turn off Instant Pot and quick-release pressure. Carefully remove lid, allowing steam to escape away from you. Using slotted spoon, transfer meatballs to plate, tent with aluminum foil, and let rest while cooking couscous. (You should have about 2 cups cooking liquid remaining in pot; add extra broth as needed to equal 2 cups.) • Using highest Sauté function, bring liquid in pot to simmer. Stir in couscous, red peppers, and lemon zest and juice. Turn off Instant Pot, cover, and let sit for 10 minutes. Fluff couscous gently with fork and transfer to serving dish. Arrange meatballs on top and drizzle with remaining ¼ cup Tahini Sauce. Sprinkle with pickled onions and remaining 2 tablespoons mint. Serve.

Lemon-Herb Chicken

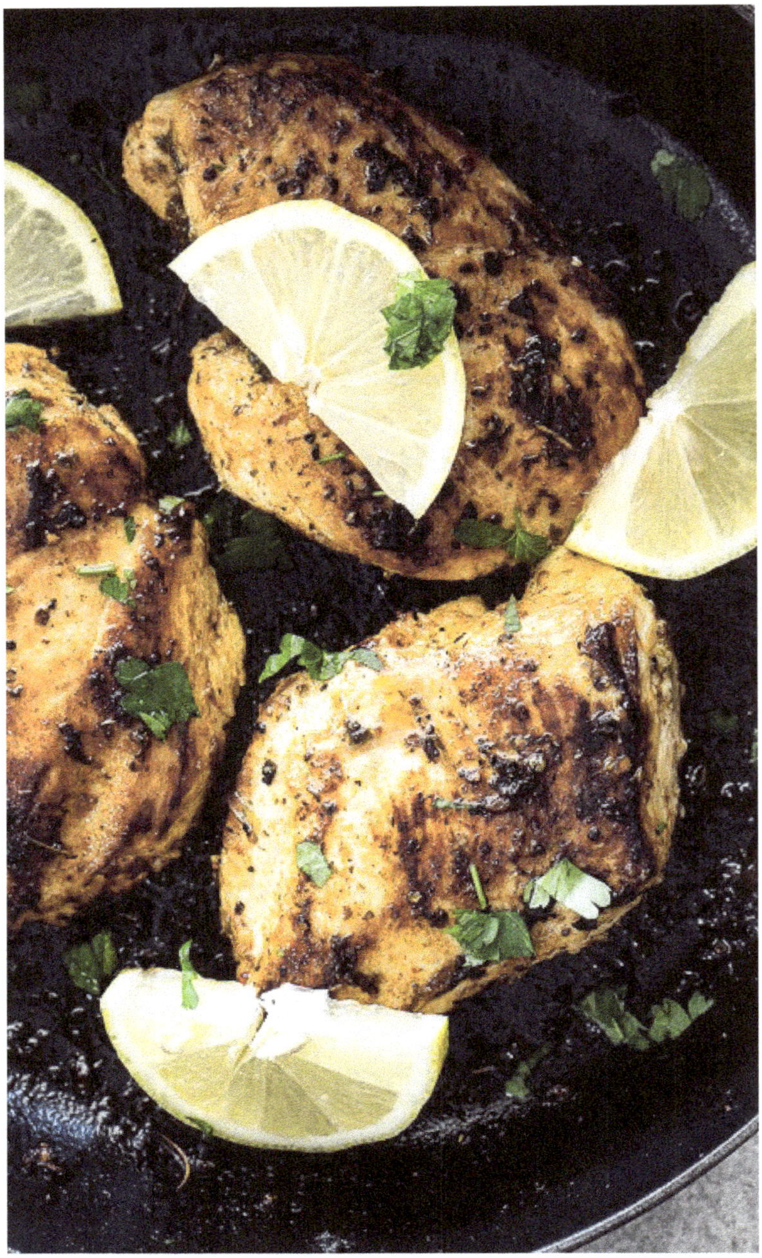

Ingredients for 4 servings:
1 Tbsp. oil 1 ½ lbs boneless, skinless chicken breasts cut into strips ½ cup Water 1 jar INSTANT POT Zesty Lemon Herb Sauce 15 oz
Directions and total time – 30-60 m • HEAT oil in Instant Pot using SAUTÉ setting on high heat. Add chicken; cook 5 min., stirring frequently. • ADD water and sauce. Do not stir. Close and lock lid. Turn Pressure Release Valve to Sealing position. • COOK 6 min. using HIGH PRESSURE COOK/MANUAL setting. When timer goes off, use Quick Pressure Release to release pressure before carefully opening lid.

BBQ Meatballs

Ingredients for 40 meatballs:

2 lbs lean ground beef ½ cup finely chopped onions ¼ cup finely chopped fresh parsley 1 tbsp minced Garlic 2 tsp LEA & PERRINS Worcestershire Sauce 1 tsp salt ½ tsp black pepper 2 eggs beaten 1 cup dry bread crumbs divided 1 jar INSTANT POT Southern BBQ Sauce divided, 15 oz ½ cup fat-free reduced-sodium beef broth

Directions and total time – 30-60 m • 1 cup water to INSTANT POT. Place trivet in pot. • Mix first 8 ingredients in large bowl just until blended. Add half the bread crumbs and 2 tbsp barbecue sauce; mix lightly. Gently mix in remaining bread crumbs. • Shape meat mixture into 40 meatballs (½ inch-1 inch) • Place half the meatballs in single layer on trivet; cover with second layer of meatballs. Close and lock lid. Turn Pressure Release Valve to Sealing position. • Cook 7 min using MANUAL/HIGH PRESSURE COOK setting. When timer goes off, use Natural Pressure Release for 5 min., then do a Quick Pressure Release to release any remaining steam. Remove lid. • Use tongs to transfer meatballs to serving bowl; cover to keep warm. Remove trivet from INSTANT POT. Discard meat juices from pot. Rinse liner, then return liner to pot. • Add beef broth and remaining barbecue sauce to pot; stir. Cook using SAUTÉ setting 3 min. or until heated through, stirring frequently. Pour over meatballs; stir to evenly coat meatballs with sauce.

Mac Cincinnati Chili

Ingredients for 4 servings:

Spice Blend: 1 tbsp sweet paprika 2 tsp ground cumin 1 ½ tsp ground cinnamon 1 tsp ground coriander 1 tsp natural cocoa powder 1 tsp mustard powder ½ tsp ground ginger ¼ tsp ground cloves ¼ tsp cayenne pepper Other Ingredients: 2 tsp cold-pressed avocado oil 2 garlic cloves minced 1 yellow onion diced, plus ¾ cup chopped, for serving 1 lb 96 percent extra-lean ground beef 2 cups low-sodium roasted beef bone broth 8 oz whole-wheat elbow pasta 14 ½ oz petite diced tomatoes and their liquid one can 1 ½ cups drained cooked kidney beans or 15 oz (1 can) kidney beans, rinsed and drained ¾ cup shredded Cheddar cheese or vegan cheese shreds, for serving yellow mustard for serving Tabasco sauce for serving

Directions and total time – 30-60 m

• To make the spice blend: In a small bowl, stir together the paprika, cumin, cinnamon, coriander, cocoa powder, mustard powder, ginger, cloves, and cayenne. • Select the Sauté setting on the Instant Pot and heat the oil and garlic for 2 minutes, until the garlic is bubbling but not browned. Add the diced onion and sauté. for about 2 minutes, until it begins to soften. Add the beef and sauté. for 3 minutes, using a wooden spoon to break up the meat as it cooks. Stir in the spice blend and sauté. for about 2 more minutes, until the beef is mostly cooked through and the spices are aromatic. • Pour in the broth, using a wooden spoon or spatula to nudge any browned bits from the bottom of the pot. Add the pasta in an even layer, using the spoon to nudge the noodles under the liquid as much as possible. It's fine if a few pieces are sticking up out of the water. Pour the tomatoes and their liquid and the kidney beans evenly over the ground beef and pasta mixture. Do not stir them in. • Secure the lid and set the Pressure Release to Sealing. Press the Cancel button to reset the cooking program, then select the Pressure Cook or Manual setting and set the cooking time for 6 minutes at high pressure. (The pot will take about 10 minutes to come up to pressure before the cooking program begins.) • When the cooking program ends, let the pressure release naturally for 5 minutes, then move the Pressure Release to Venting to release any remaining steam. Open the pot and stir the chili mac to combine. Let sit for 5 minutes, then stir once more.

Salmon with Spinach and Potatoes
Ingredients for 4 servings:
1 lb small red potatoes quartered 1 cup Water 1 ¼ tsp salt divided ¾ tsp black pepper divided 4 salmon filets 5-ounces each ¼ tsp sweet paprika ½ tsp lemon zest 4 garlic cloves minced 2 tbsp avocado oil 4 cups packed baby spinach 4 lemon wedges
Directions and total time – 15-30 m
• Place the potatoes in the inner pot and add 1 cup water, ¼ teaspoon salt, and ¼ teaspoon pepper. Place a steam rack on top of the potatoes. • On top of the salmon add the paprika, lemon zest, ½ teaspoon salt, and ¼ teaspoon pepper and place the salmon on top of the steam rack. Secure the lid. • Press the Manual or Pressure Cook button and adjust the time to 3 minutes. • When the timer beeps, let pressure release naturally until float valve drops and then unlock lid. • Remove the salmon and steam rack from the pot and set aside. • Press the Sauté button and cook the potatoes 1 minute. Add the garlic and cook an additional 2 minutes, stirring frequently. Stir in the oil and the remaining salt and pepper. Use a fork to gently mash the potatoes to achieve a chunky texture. Press the Cancel button. • Add the spinach and stir until wilted, about 1–2 minutes. Serve the salmon and potato and spinach mixture with the lemon wedges.

Pork Tenderloin with Sriracha and Honey
Ingredients for 2-4 servings:
1 lb pork tenderloin (or can use up to 1 ½ lbs) 2 tbsp honey 2 tbsp sriracha hot sauce or to taste 1 ½ tsp kosher salt
Directions and total time – 30-60 m
• Insert the spit through the center of the pork tenderloin. Use a pointed metal skewer to make an initial hole if needed. Thread the rotisserie forks from each side and tighten the screws to hold the pork firmly in place. • In a small bowl, combine the honey, sriracha and salt. Brush evenly over the pork tenderloin. • Place the drip pan in the bottom of the cooking chamber. Using the display panel, select AIRFRY, then adjust the temperature to 350°F and the time to 20 minutes, then touch START. • When the display indicates "Add Food" use the rotisserie fetch tool to lift the spit into the cooking chamber, using the red rotisserie release lever to secure the ends of the spit. Close the door and touch ROTATE.

Oregano Scallops Alfredo
Ingredients for 4 servings:
1 ¾ cups alfredo sauce 16 ouncejar 2 ½ cups chicken or vegetable broth ½ tsp dried oregano ½ tsp garlic powder ½ tsp red pepper flakes 12 oz regular no-yolk, or gluten-free dried egg noodles 1 lb frozen bay scallops
Directions and total time – 30-60 m • Put 1 ½ cups of the alfredo sauce in an Instant Pot. Stir in the broth, oregano, garlic powder, and red pepper flakes until smooth. Stir in the noodles, then set the block of frozen scallops right on top. Lock the lid onto the pot. • Option 1 Max Pressure Cooker Press Pressure cook on Max pressure for 3 minutes with the Keep Warm setting off. • Option 2 All Pressure Cookers Press Meat/Stew or Pressure cook (Manual) on High pressure for 4 minutes with the Keep Warm setting off. • When the machine has finished cooking, turn it off and let its pressure return to normal naturally for 1 minute. Then use the quick-release method to get rid of any residual pressure in the pot. • Unlatch the lid and open the cooker. Stir in the remaining ¼ cup alfredo sauce. Set the lid askew over the pot and let sit for a couple of minutes so the noodles continue to absorb some of the liquid. Serve hot.

Burrito Shredded Chicken and Rice Bowl

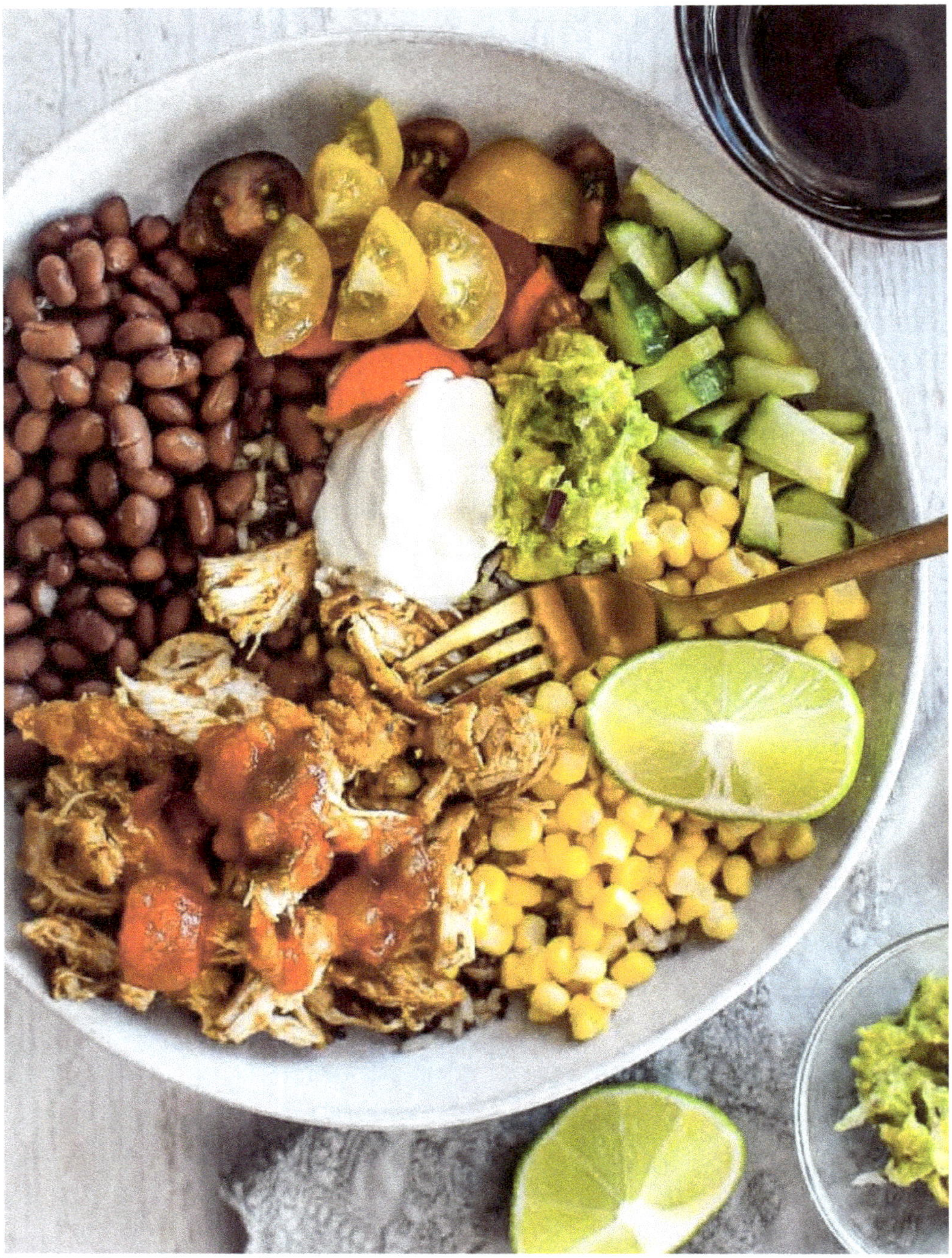

Ingredients for 6 servings:

2 tbsp extra-virgin olive oil 2 lbs boneless, skinless chicken breasts 5 - 6 chicken breasts 1 tsp ground cumin ¼ tsp cayenne pepper or taco seasoning 1 medium red or white onion chopped 4 oz green chiles chopped or diced 1 can 1 ½ cups low-sodium chicken broth 15 oz pinto beans drained and rinsed 1 can 3 cups cooked brown rice 2 medium avocados pitted and sliced, for garnish fresh chopped cilantro for garnish Sliced jalapeño for garnish prepared salsa for garnish (optional)

Directions and total time – 30-60 m • Select Sauté and add the olive oil to the inner pot. Once the oil is hot, place the chicken breasts in the pot and brown them for 2 minutes per side. • Press Cancel and add the cumin, cayenne pepper, onion, green chiles, and chicken broth. Using a wooden spoon, scrape up any browned bits stuck to the bottom of the pot. • Lock the lid into place. Select Pressure Cook or Manual; set the pressure to High and the time to 15 minutes. Make sure the steam release knob is in the sealed position. After cooking, naturally release the pressure for 10 minutes, then quick release any remaining pressure. • Unlock and remove the lid. Use a slotted spoon to transfer the chicken to a cutting board. Shred the chicken using two forks, and then add it back to the pot. Add the pinto beans and stir the ingredients to combine. • Serve immediately, or place the chicken and rice in an airtight container and refrigerate for up to 4 days or freeze for up to 2 months. • When ready to serve, divide the rice among six bowls and ladle the chicken mixture on top. Garnish each bowl with 2 slices of fresh avocado, cilantro, jalapeño, and a spoonful of salsa (if using).

Savory Pie

Ingredients for 4-6 servings:

Beef Mixture: 1 lb ground beef preferably 93% lean 1 onion finely diced 1 ½ cups frozen peas and carrots mixture 1 cup mushrooms roughly chopped 2 tbsp Worcestershire sauce 1 tsp salt 1 tsp pepper After Saute: 2 tbsp butter 2 tbsp flour ½ cup beef broth Potato Mixture: 1 cup Water 1 ½ lbs russet potatoes peeled and cut into 1 inch cubes 2 tbsp butter 1 egg beaten 1 tsp kosher salt 1 tsp garlic powder To Finish: 1 cup shredded Cheddar cheese

Directions and total time – 30-60 m • Add ground beef and onion to the Instant Pot. Using the display panel select the SAUTE function. • Cook and stir until no pink remains. Drain any liquids. • Add remaining Beef Mixture ingredients and stir to combine. • In a small bowl, melt >2 tbsp butter. Whisk in flour and beef broth until smooth. Add to pot and stir to combine. • Cook and stir for 3-4 minutes, until sauce begins to thicken. • Transfer the beef mixture to a 1 ½ qt Instant Pot-friendly casserole and cover to keep warm. • Rinse out the pot, then combine 1 cup water and cubed potatoes in the pot. • Turn the pot off by selecting CANCEL, then secure the lid, making sure the vent is closed. • Using the display panel select the MANUAL or PRESSURE COOK function. Use the +/- keys and program the Instant Pot for 8 minutes. • When the time is up, quick-release the pressure. • Add remaining Potato Mixture ingredients to the pot and mash to desired consistency. • Top the beef mixture evenly with the mashed potatoes. Cover the casserole with foil. • Rinse out the pot, then add 1 ½ cups of water and the steam rack. • Carefully lower the casserole onto the rack, then secure the lid, making sure the vent is closed. • Using the display panel select the MANUAL or PRESSURE COOK function. Use the +/- keys and program the Instant Pot for 10 minutes. • When the time is up, quick-release the pressure. • Carefully remove the dish from the pot, top with cheese and let rest for 10 minutes before serving. • (Optional) Set under broiler for 5-7 minutes until cheese is lightly browned.

Corned Beef with Cabbage
Ingredients for 6 servings:
3 carrots, peeled and cut into 3-inch pieces 1 yellow onion, peeled and quartered ½ pound small potatoes, halved 1 corned beef brisket (about 3 pounds), plus pickling spice packet or 1 tablespoon pickling spice 2 8-ounce beers 6 sprigs fresh thyme ½ head Savoy cabbage, cut into 1 ½-inch wedges ½ cup sour cream 3-4 tablespoons prepared horseradish, to taste
Directions and total time – more than 2 h To Cook in the Slow Cooker: • In a 5-to-6-quart slow cooker, place the carrots, onion and potatoes. Place corned beef, fat side up, on top of the vegetables and sprinkle with pickling spice. Pour the beers over the vegetables and brisket. Sprinkle with the sprigs of fresh thyme. Cover and cook on high until corned beef is tender, 5-6 hours or 10-12 hours on low. • Arrange cabbage over corned beef, cover, and continue cooking until cabbage is tender, 45 min to 1 hour (or 1 ½ to 2 hours on low). Thinly slice the corned beef against the grain and serve with the vegetables and cooking liquid with the horseradish sauce. To Cook in the Instant Pot: • Cut the corned beef into 2-3 chunks so it cooks faster and more evenly. Add to the insert of a 6 quart Instant Pot with the fat cap up. Layer with the onion, spices, thyme and beer. Cook on HIGH pressure for 90 minutes then do a quick release. • Add the potatoes, carrots and cabbage to the insert, close, and set to HIGH pressure for another 5 minutes. Natural release for 5 minutes, cut, and serve. For the Horseradish Sauce: • Mix the sour cream and horseradish together in a small bowl. Refrigerate for up to 1 week.

Beef and Barley Soup

Ingredients for 6-8 servings: 1 ½ pounds stew meat salt and pepper 2 tablespoons oil 10 baby bella mushrooms, quartered 3 cups mirepoix (just a combination of chopped onion, celery, and carrots) 6-8 cloves garlic, minced 6 cups low sodium beef broth (or vegetable) 1 cup water 2 bay leaves ½ teaspoon dried thyme 1 large potato, shredded (using a food processor or grater) ⅔ cup pearl barley, rinsed

Directions and total time – 1-2 h • Season the stew meat with a good pinch of salt and pepper. Heat 1 tablespoon of oil in a large pot or in the instant pot over medium-high heat. Add ½ the stew meat and brown on all sides for about 2-3 minutes total. Remove meat to a plate and repeat with the second batch and the second tablespoon of oil. • Add the mushroom to the pot and brown the mushrooms for 1-2 minutes or until they start picking up the brown bits left behind by the meat. Remove the mushrooms to the same plate as the stew meat. • If needed, add a little more oil to the pot and the mirepoix mix. Cook the veggies for 4-5 minutes or until the onions soften and become translucent. Add the garlic and cook for an additional 30 seconds • Add the stew meat, mushrooms, bay leaves, dried thyme, water, and beef broth the to sautéed veggies in the instant pot, cover and pressure cook the meat for 13-16 minutes depending on the size of the stew meat. Allow the pressure to release before removing the lid.

Softly Turkey Breast

Ingredients for 6-8 servings: 7 lb bone-in turkey breast 3 tbsp butter softened ½ tsp paprika ¼ tsp garlic powder ½ tsp salt 1 ½ cups chicken broth or water 1 small onion quartered 2 small celery stalks cut in half 2 tbsp cornstarch Plus additional 1 tsp

Directions and total time – 30-60 m • If the turkey breast is frozen, let it thaw in refrigerator for 3 days in the wrapping it came in. Remove the gravy mix and giblets from the cavity, if any are present. Rinse the turkey breast and let it drain in a colander. Pat it dry with paper towels. Loosen the skin on top of the breast with your fingers and a knife but do not cut it off. • Combine butter, herb seasoning, and salt in a small bowl. Using fingertips, spread about 2 tbsp of the mixture up under the skin and onto the turkey breast. Lay the skin over the mixture then spread the remaining mixture on top of the skin. • Place the trivet in the Instant Pot pan and pour in the chicken broth. • If the turkey breast has a cavity to place the onion and celery under the breast, place it there. If it is open, just place them in the Instant Pot pan and place the turkey breast, breast side up. • Place lid on Instant Pot and set valve to "sealing". Press "Pressure Cook"/ "Manual" button, then -/+ button to 32 minutes on High Pressure. It will take about 12 to 20 minutes to come to pressure, cook 32 minutes, then when it beeps, let it release pressure naturally (don't touch sealing valve) for 20 minutes. If it hasn't release all the pressure, switch to "venting". Carefully open the lid away from your face when floating valve drops. • Preheat broiler. Remove the turkey with two large metal spatulas or spoons. Forks will release all the turkey juices! Place it on a foil-lined baking sheet and broil it 3 to 5 inches from the broiler for 3 to 5 minutes or just until skin in golden brown. • Measure 2 cups of turkey drippings in the Instant Pot pan. Discard any remaining liquid, onion and celery (I actually save them for soup later). Combine 1 tbsp water and cornstarch in a custard dish then pour into turkey drippings. Turn Instant Pot "Saute" button on. Cook the gravy, stirring constantly about 8 minutes or until slightly thickened.

Pork Meatball with Cream Sauce

Ingredients for 6 servings:

1 ¼ pounds ground pork 2 strips bacon minced 1 egg mixed ½ medium onion minced 2 tablespoons almond flour 1 clove garlic minced ¼ teaspoon pepper cracked ½ teaspoon sea salt 1 tablespoon tomato paste 1 tablespoon liquid aminos or tamari or soy sauce 2 tablespoons avocado oil or coconut oil 1 ½ cups Water or chicken stock 2 tablespoons butter salted, melted ½ teaspoon xanthan gum optional ⅔ cup heavy cream 33% ½ teaspoon sea salt ¼ teaspoon cracked pepper

Directions and total time – 30-60 m

• In a bowl mix the ground pork, bacon, egg, onion, almond flour, garlic, cracked pepper, sea salt and liquid aminos together. • Take 2 tablespoons of the meatball mixture and shape into a ball using wet hands. Place on a flat surface such as a cookie sheet. • Continue shaping meatballs. Makes about 24 weighing about 1 ounce each. • Press Sauté on the Instant Pot. Once display reads "hot", add avocado oil. • Carefully place half the meatballs into pot evenly spaced. After two minutes, turn them over. • After a minute, roll them onto a side. After another minute, remove and set aside on a plate. • Continue from step 5 to 7 with second batch of meat balls. • Once the second batch of meat balls are brown, remove and place with first batch. • Deglaze pot with water or chicken stock, be sure to scrape as much of the bits off the sides and bottom of the pan. • Add the meatballs back into the pot along with any drippings. Press cancel on the Instant Pot to stop Sauté. • Close lid and lock. Seal the pressure release valve. Press Manual and adjust to high pressure. Set time for 7 minutes to cook. • In the meantime, whisk xanthan gum into melted butter. • After cooking time is complete, press Cancel and Quick Release the pressure release valve. Unlock and open the lid. Remove the meatballs and set aside. • Press Sauté. Whisk in butter with xanthan gum into water/stock. • Next whisk in cream, salt and pepper in the Instant Pot. Let the sauce heat for 2 minutes while whisking. • Add the meatballs along with any drippings into the sauce and stir around to coat. • Ladle the meatballs with sauce into a bowl.

Chipotle Brisket

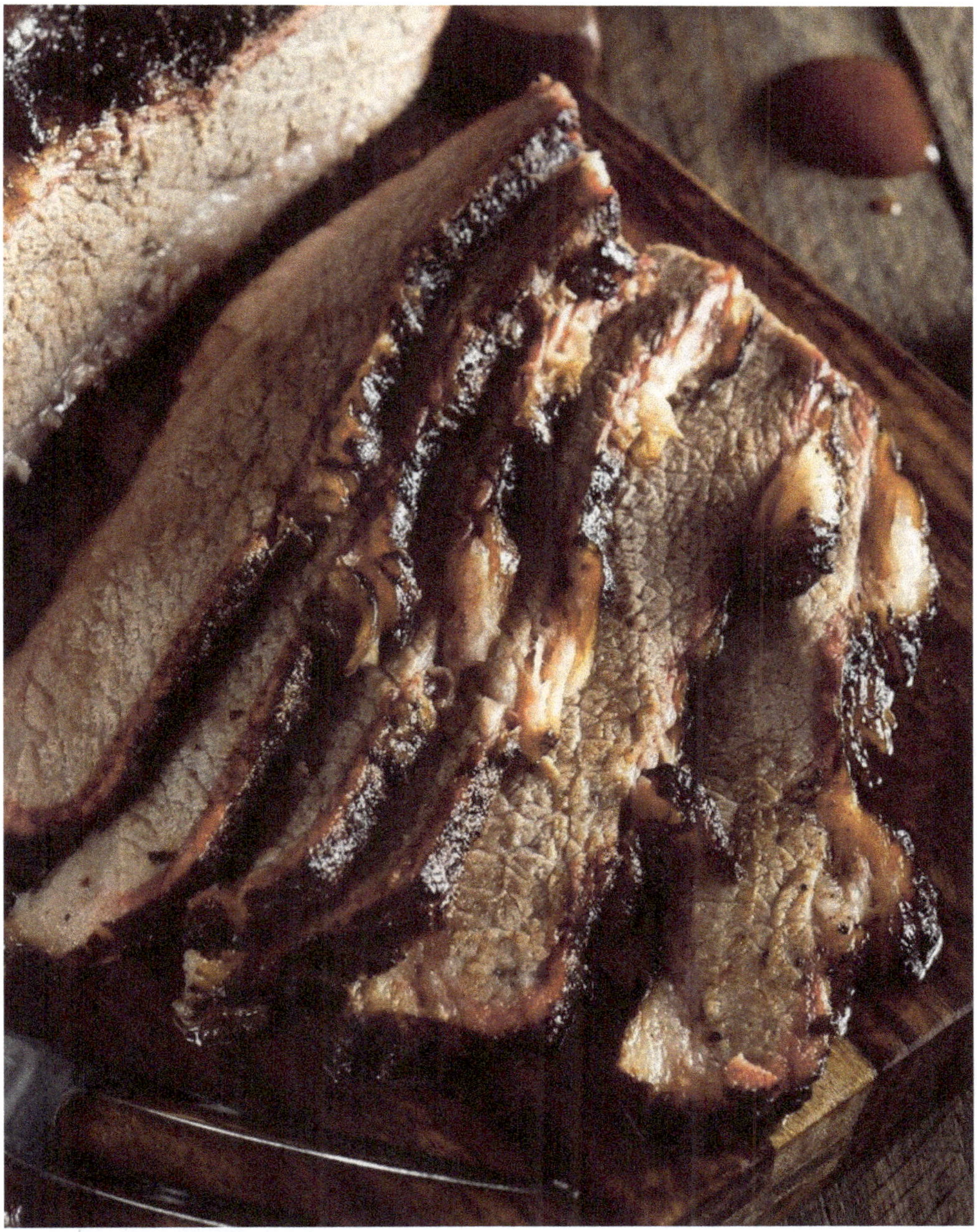

Ingredients for 4-6 servings:

3 ½ pounds beef brisket 1 tablespoons bacon fat 2 tablespoons chipotle powder 1 cup water 1 teaspoons fine sea salt ¼ cup chopped cilantro, for garnish1 tablespoon sesame oil

Directions and total time – 1-2 h

• Cut brisket into 4 equal pieces. • Add bacon fat to Instant Pot and turn to "saute." • Season brisket with chipotle powder by making sure it's applied liberally and rubbed into all sides. Once the fat is melted, add the beef to Instant Pot in two batches, searing brisket for 2-3 minutes per side until browned. Note: searing the beef all at once will cause overcrowding and will prevent the beef from browning nicely. • Once all beef is browned, add all pieces back to the pot along with water. • Close the instant pot, making sure the valve is set to "sealing" rather than "venting." Hit the "meat/stew" button and adjust to cook for 70 minutes. • Once the brisket is finished cooking, let the Instant pot release pressure naturally (about 15 minutes) until the lid easily opens. • Slice the beef against the grain and serve. Garnish with sea salt and cilantro, if desired.

Barbecue Spare Ribs
(Ready in about 35 minutes | Servings 8)
Per serving: 444 Calories; 33g Fat; 4.4g Carbs; 32.5g Protein; 1.7g Sugars
Ingredients
3 pounds spare ribs Sea salt and ground black pepper, to taste 1/2 teaspoon granulated garlic 1 teaspoon cayenne pepper For the sauce: 3/4 cup tomato puree A few drops of stevia 1 tablespoon balsamic vinegar 1/3 cup broth 1 cup water 1/3 teaspoon liquid smoke 1/2 teaspoon ground cloves
Directions
Season the ribs with salt, black pepper, garlic, and cayenne pepper. Add the spare ribs to the Instant Pot. Combine the ingredients for the sauce; whisk until everything is well mixed. Pour this sauce mixture over the spare ribs. Secure the lid. Choose the "Meat/Stew" setting and cook for 30 minutes under High pressure. Once cooking is complete, use a natural pressure release; carefully remove the lid. You can thicken the cooking liquid with a tablespoon or two of flaxseed meal if desired. Enjoy!

Family Pork Roast
(Ready in about 30 minutes | Servings 6)
Per serving: 329 Calories; 18.2g Fat; 0g Carbs; 38.7g Protein; 0g Sugars
Ingredients
2 teaspoons peanut oil 2 pounds pork tenderloin 1 cup beef bone broth 2 bay leaves 1 teaspoon mixed peppercorns
Directions
Massage the peanut oil into the pork. Press the "Sauté" button to heat up the Instant Pot. Heat the oil and sear the meat for 2 to 3 minute on both sides. Add the broth, bay leaves and mixed peppercorns to the Instant Pot. Secure the lid. Choose the "Meat/Stew" setting and cook for 20 minutes under High pressure. Once cooking is complete, use a natural pressure release; carefully remove the lid. Serve over cauli rice. Bon appétit!

Pork Meatballs alla Parmigiana
(Ready in about 15 minutes | Servings 6)
Per serving: 356 Calories; 17.2g Fat; 5.6g Carbs; 44.7g Protein; 1.5g Sugars

Ingredients

2 pounds lean ground pork 1 teaspoon red pepper flakes, crushed 1 cup grated parmesan cheese 1/4 cup pork rinds, crushed 1 egg 1 teaspoon garlic paste 2 tablespoons scallions, chopped Seasoned salt and ground black pepper, to taste 1 teaspoon shallot powder 1/2 teaspoon dried basil 1/2 teaspoon dried sage, crushed 1/4 cup beef bone broth 1 tablespoon sesame oil 2 cups keto tomato sauce 4 ounces mozzarella cheese, slices

Directions

In a mixing bowl, thoroughly combine ground pork, red pepper, parmesan cheese, pork rinds, egg, garlic paste, scallions, aromatics, and beef bone broth. Mix to combine well. Now, shape the mixture into 2-inch meatballs. Press the "Sauté" button to heat up the Instant Pot. Heat the oil until sizzling. Now, sear the meatballs until delicately browned. Pour the tomato sauce over the meatballs. Secure the lid. Choose the "Manual" setting and cook for 8 minutes under High pressure. Once cooking is complete, use a quick pressure release; carefully remove the lid. Afterwards, top the meatballs with mozzarella slices and broil them until mozzarella is golden. Bon appétit!

Tender Pulled Pork
(Ready in about 55 minutes | Servings 6)
Per serving: 434 Calories; 29.1g Fat; 1.5g Carbs; 38.6g Protein; 0.4g Sugars
Ingredients
2 pounds pork butt Celery salt and ground black pepper, to your liking 1 tablespoon lard 4 cloves garlic, smashed 1/2 teaspoon caraway seeds 1/2 teaspoon mustard seeds 1 bay leaf 1 cup beef bone broth 1 tablespoon chile powder 1 teaspoon cayenne pepper 1/2 teaspoon hot Hungarian paprika 1/2 teaspoon onion powder
Directions
Season the pork butt with salt and ground black pepper. Press the "Sauté" button to heat up the Instant Pot. Melt the lard and brown the pork on all sides. Add the remaining ingredients. Secure the lid. Choose the "Manual" setting and cook for 50 minutes under High pressure. Once cooking is complete, use a natural pressure release; carefully remove the lid. Shred the meat with two forks and serve with keto bread rolls. Bon appétit!

Sloppy Joes with Homemade Oopsies
(Ready in about 35 minutes | Servings 4)
Per serving: 524 Calories; 45g Fat; 5.5g Carbs; 27.8g Protein; 1.9g Sugars

Ingredients

Sloppy Joes 1 tablespoon olive oil 1 pound lean ground pork 1/2 yellow onion, chopped 2 cloves garlic, minced 1 tomato, puréed 1 teaspoon stone ground mustard 1 tablespoon coconut aminos 1 cup roasted vegetable broth Sea salt and ground black pepper, to taste Oopsies: 2 eggs, separated yolks and whites 1/4 teaspoon sea salt 3 ounces cream cheese 1/4 teaspoon baking powder

Directions

Press the "Sauté" button to heat up the Instant Pot. Heat the oil until sizzling. Brown the ground pork for 2 to 3 minutes, crumbling with a fork. Add the other ingredients for Sloppy Joes and stir to combine well. Secure the lid. Choose the "Manual" setting and cook for 5 minutes under High pressure. Once cooking is complete, use a quick pressure release; carefully remove the lid. To make your oopsies, beat the egg whites together with salt until very firm peaks form. In another bowl, thoroughly combine the egg yolks with cream cheese. Now, add the baking powder and stir well. Next, fold the egg white mixture into the egg yolk mixture. Divide the mixture into 6 oopsies and transfer them to a silicon sheet. Bake in the preheated oven at 290 degrees F for about 23 minutes. Serve Sloppy Joes between 2 oopsies and enjoy!

Za'atar-Rubbed Pork Shank

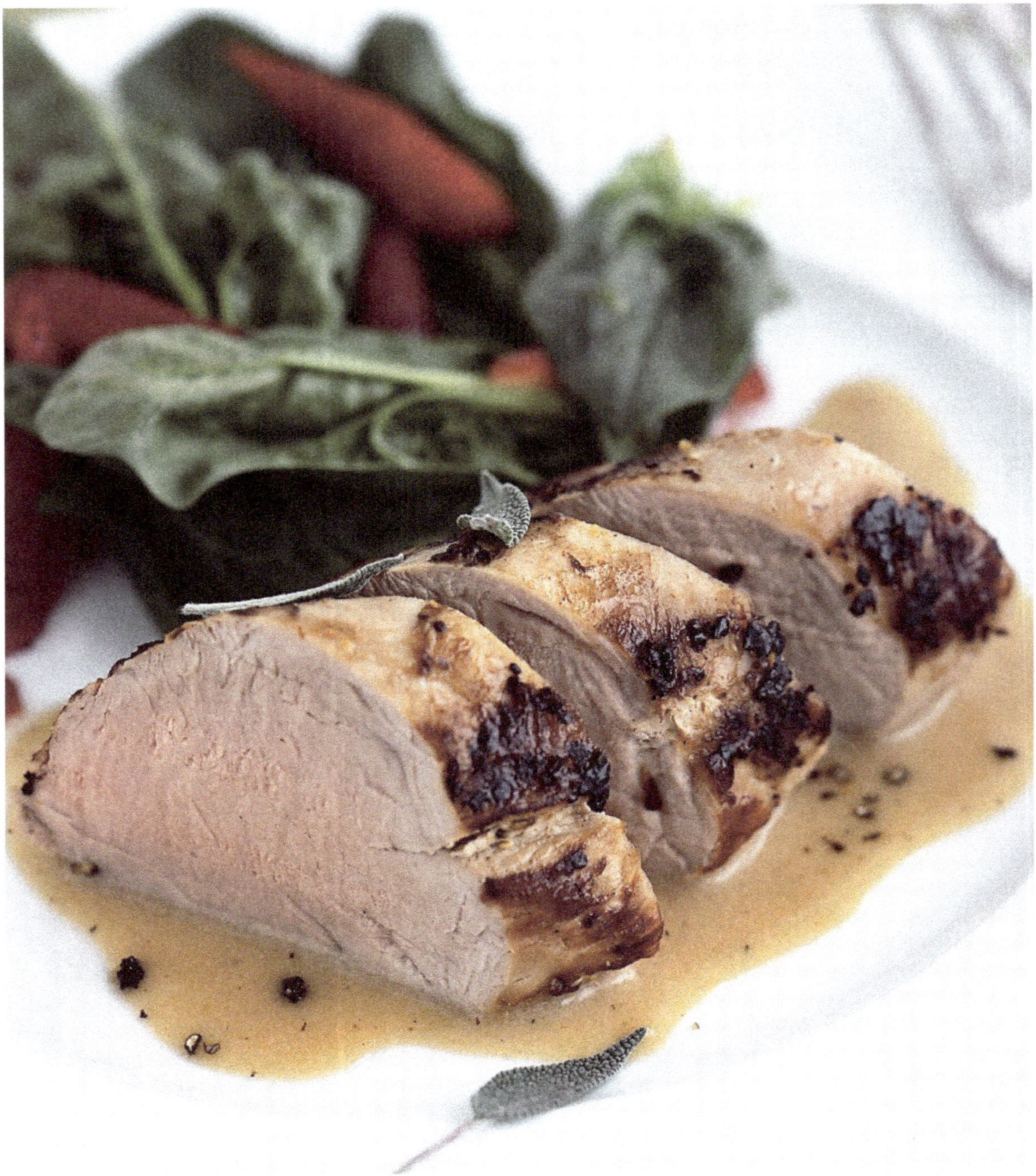

(Ready in about 45 minutes | Servings 6)
Per serving: 328 Calories; 18.1g Fat; 9g Carbs; 30.6g Protein; 2.6g Sugars
Ingredients
1 ½ pounds pork shank Seasoned salt and ground black pepper, to taste 2 tablespoons za'atar 1 tablespoon olive oil 1 medium-sized leek, sliced 2 garlic cloves, smashed 1 carrot, chopped 1 parsnip, chopped 1 celery with leaves,

chopped 1 tablespoon dark soy sauce 1/2 teaspoon mustard powder 1 cup beef bone broth 1 tablespoon flaxseed meal

Directions Generously season the pork shank with salt and black pepper. Now, sprinkle with za'atar on all sides. Press the "Sauté" button to heat up the Instant Pot. Heat the olive oil. Once hot, sear the pork shank for 2 to 4 minute per side; reserve. Now, sauté leeks in pan drippings for 3 minutes. After that, add the garlic, carrot parsnip, celery with leaves, soy sauce, mustard powder, and broth. Add the pork shank back to the Instant Pot. Secure the lid. Choose the "Meat/Stew" setting and cook for 35 minutes under High pressure. Once cooking is complete, use a natural pressure release; carefully remove the lid. Mix flaxseed meal with 1 tablespoon of water. Add this slurry to the Instant Pot. Press the "Sauté" button again to thicken the cooking liquid. Serve warm.

Greek-Style Pork Stew
(Ready in about 15 minutes | Servings 8)
Per serving: 249 Calories; 10.1g Fat; 5.1g Carbs; 31.2g Protein; 2.7g Sugars

Ingredients

1 tablespoon olive oil 2 ½ pounds pork stew meat, cubed 1 red onion, chopped 4 cloves garlic, peeled 1 bell pepper, chopped 2 tablespoons Greek red wine 1 cup beef bone broth 1 star anise Coarse sea salt and ground black pepper, to taste 1 teaspoon dried basil 1 teaspoon dried oregano 1/2 teaspoon dried dill weed 1 (14.5-ounce) can diced tomatoes 2 tablespoons fresh basil leaves, snipped

Directions

Press the "Sauté" button to heat up the Instant Pot. Heat the olive oil and sauté the meat until browned; reserve. Then, in pan drippings, cook the onion, garlic, and bell pepper until softened. Add red wine to deglaze the pan. Add beef bone broth, star anise, sea salt, black pepper, dried basil, oregano, dill and canned tomatoes. Secure the lid. Choose the "Manual" setting and cook for 10 minutes under High pressure. Once cooking is complete, use a quick pressure release; carefully remove the lid. Ladle into individual bowls and serve garnished with fresh basil leaves. Bon appétit!

Pork Cutlets with Porcini Mushroom Sauce
(Ready in about 15 minutes | Servings 4)
Per serving: 412 Calories; 25.4g Fat; 2.1g Carbs; 41.5g Protein; 0.8g Sugars

Ingredients

2 teaspoons olive oil 4 pork cutlets Seasoned salt to taste 1/2 teaspoon ground black pepper 1/2 teaspoon cayenne pepper 1/2 cup scallions, chopped 1 cup Porcini mushrooms, thinly sliced 1 teaspoon roasted garlic paste 1 bay leaf 1 cup broth, preferably homemade 1 tablespoon arrowroot powder + 1 tablespoon water 1/2 cup heavy cream

Directions

Press the "Sauté" button to heat up the Instant Pot; add olive oil. Now, sear the pork cutlets until delicately browned on both sides. Season with salt, black pepper, and cayenne pepper. Then, add the scallions, mushrooms, garlic paste, bay leaf, and broth to the Instant Pot. Secure the lid. Choose the "Manual" setting and cook for 10 minutes under High pressure. Once cooking is complete, use a quick pressure release; carefully remove the lid. Now, whisk the arrowroot powder with 1 tablespoon of water in a small mixing bowl. Ad this slurry along with heavy cream to the cooking liquid. Press the "Sauté" button again to thicken the cooking liquid. Serve this sauce over pork cutlets.

Pork Roast with Avocado and Garlic Mayo
(Ready in about 35 minutes | Servings 6
Per serving: 390 Calories; 22.4g Fat; 3g Carbs; 42.1g Protein; 0.7g Sugars
Ingredients
Pork Roast: 1 tablespoon lard, melted 2 pounds pork roast 1 cup chicken stock 1/2 cup shallots, chopped 1 celery rib, chopped 1 tablespoon fish sauce 1 tablespoon coconut aminos 1/4 teaspoon ground black pepper Sea salt, to your liking Avocado and Garlic Mayo: 1/3 cup mayonnaise 1/2 avocado, pitted and peeled 2 garlic cloves, pressed 1 teaspoon lemon juice
Directions
Press the "Sauté" button to heat up the Instant Pot. Melt the lard and brown pork roast for 2 to 4 minutes. Now, add the pork roast, chicken stock, shallots, celery, fish, sauce, coconut aminos, black pepper, and sea salt to the Instant Pot. Secure the lid. Choose the "Manual" setting and cook for 30 minutes under High pressure. Once cooking is complete, use a natural pressure release; carefully remove the lid. In the meantime, mix all ingredients for the mayonnaise in your food processor or blender. Cut pork roast into slices and serve with Avocado and Garlic Mayo on the side. Bon appétit!

Pork Loin with Goat-Cheese Sauce
(Ready in about 20 minutes | Servings 6
Per serving: 449 Calories; 27.5g Fat; 4.5g Carbs; 43.8g Protein; 2.3g Sugars

Ingredients

1 tablespoon grapeseed oil 2 pounds pork loin, sliced 2 garlic cloves, pressed 1 red onion, chopped 1 bell pepper, chopped 1 jalapeño pepper, finely chopped 1/2 cup vegetable stock 1/2 cup double cream 2 ounces Ricotta cheese 1/2 cup goat cheese 1/2 teaspoon dried basil 1/2 teaspoon dried marjoram 1/2 teaspoon celery seeds 1/3 teaspoon pepper Sea salt, to your liking

Directions

Press the "Sauté" button to heat up the Instant Pot. Heat the oil until sizzling. Now, sear the pork loin until slightly browned on both sides, approximately 3 minutes. Add the garlic, onion, pepper, and vegetable stock to the Instant Pot. Secure the lid. Choose the "Manual" setting and cook for 12 minutes under High pressure. Once cooking is complete, use a natural pressure release; carefully remove the lid. Next, add the remaining ingredients and let it cook in the residual heat or until cheese is melted. Add pork chops back to the cheese sauce and serve. Bon appétit!

Easy Curried Pork Steak

(Ready in about 15 minutes | Servings 6

Per serving: 362 Calories; 25.2g Fat; 2.2g Carbs; 29.6g Protein; 0.9g Sugars

Ingredients

1/2 teaspoon mustard seeds 1 teaspoon fennel seeds 1 teaspoon cumin seeds 2 chili peppers, seeded and minced 1/2 teaspoon ground bay leaf 1 teaspoon mixed peppercorns 1 tablespoon sesame oil 1 ½ pounds pork steak, sliced 1 cup chicken broth 2 tablespoons scallions, chopped 2 cloves garlic, finely minced 1 teaspoon fresh ginger, grated 1 teaspoon curry powder 2 tablespoons balsamic vinegar 3 tablespoons coconut cream 1/4 teaspoon ground black pepper 1/4 teaspoon red pepper flakes, crushed Sea salt, to taste

Directions

Heat a cast-iron skillet over medium-high heat. Once hot, roast mustard seeds, fennel seeds, cumin, peppers, ground bay leaf and peppercorns until aromatic. Press the "Sauté" button to heat up the Instant Pot. Heat the sesame oil until sizzling. Then, sear pork steak until delicately browned. Add the remaining ingredients, including roasted seasonings; stir well. Add vegetable broth and secure the lid. Choose the "Manual" setting and cook for 8 minutes under High pressure. Once cooking is complete, use a quick pressure release; carefully remove the lid. Ladle into individual serving bowls and enjoy!

Beer Braised Boston-Style Butt

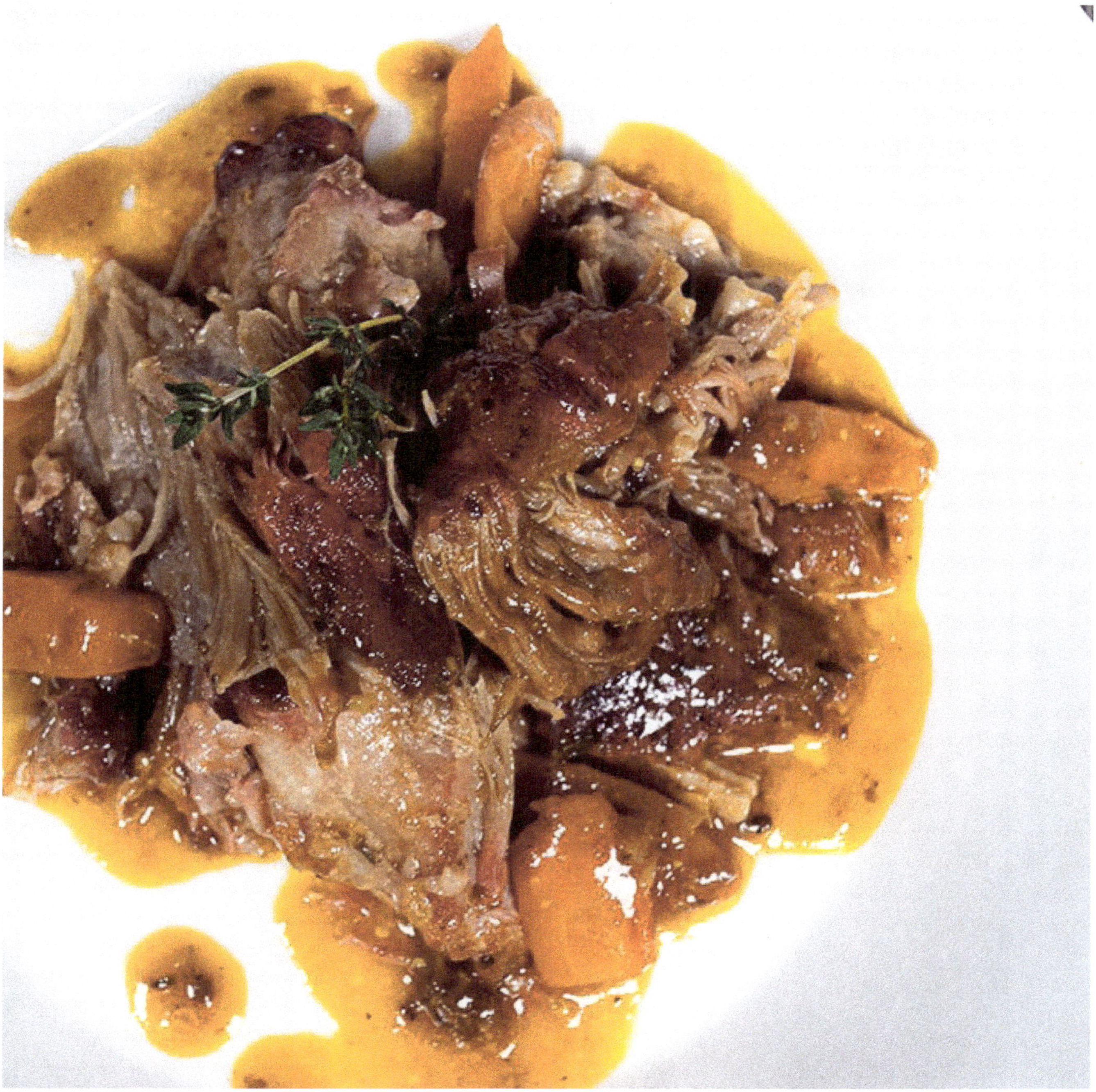

(Ready in about 55 minutes | Servings 4)
Per serving: 330 Calories; 13.1g Fat; 2.1g Carbs; 48.4g Protein; 0.4g Sugars

Ingredients

1 tablespoon lard 1 pound Boston-style butt 1/2 cup leeks, chopped 1/4 cup water 1/4 cup beer 1/2 cup chicken stock 1/4 teaspoon ground black pepper Sea salt, to taste A pinch of grated nutmeg

Directions

Press the "Sauté" button to heat up the Instant Pot. Once hot, melt the lard. Cook Boston-style butt for 2 to 3 minutes on each side; reserve. Now, sauté the leeks until fragrant; add a splash of chicken stock to deglaze the pan. Add the other ingredients and stir to combine. Secure the lid. Choose the "Manual" setting and cook for 50 minutes under High pressure. Once cooking is complete, use a natural pressure release; carefully remove the lid. Serve immediately. Enjoy!

Japanese-Style Sirloin Pork Roast
(Ready in about 2 hours 35 minutes | Servings 4)
Per serving: 364 Calories; 13.8g Fat; 4g Carbs; 53.1g Protein; 1.2g Sugars
Ingredients
1 ½ pounds sirloin pork roast Salt and ground black pepper, to taste 1/2 cup leeks, sliced 2 garlic cloves, minced 1 tablespoon Shoyu sauce 2 tablespoons Ryorishu 1 tablespoon Mirin 2 teaspoons sesame oil 6 drops Stevia liquid concentrate 1 teaspoon cayenne pepper 1 cup water 2 tablespoons black sesame seeds 2 tablespoons fresh chives, chopped
Directions
Generously season the sirloin pork roast with sea salt and ground black pepper. In a mixing bowl, thoroughly combine the leeks, garlic, Shoyu sauce, Ryorishu, mirin, sesame oil, Stevia, cayenne pepper, and water. Place the pork in a mixing bowl and let it marinate for 2 hours in your refrigerator. Place the pork and 1 cup of marinade in the Instant Pot. Secure the lid. Choose the "Meat/Stew" setting and cook for 30 minutes at High pressure. Once cooking is complete, use a natural pressure release; carefully remove the lid. Take the pork out of the Instant Pot. Then, press the "Sauté" button; add the remaining marinade. Let the cooking liquid cook until it has reduced and thickened. Slice the sirloin pork roast and place on individual serving plates. Spoon the sauce over the meat; garnish with sesame seeds and fresh chives. Bon appétit!

Pork and Bacon Chowder
(Ready in about 30 minutes | Servings 4)
Per serving: 361 Calories; 19.6g Fat; 8.2g Carbs; 37.8g Protein; 3.7g Sugars

Ingredients

1/2 pound bacon 1/2 pound pork stew meat 2 tablespoons butter 1/2 cup yellow onions, chopped 1 celery with leaves, chopped 2 garlic cloves, minced 1 cup white mushrooms, sliced 1/2 teaspoon dried rosemary 1/2 teaspoon dried thyme Sea salt, to taste 1/2 teaspoon ground black pepper 1/2 teaspoon cayenne pepper A pinch of hot paprika A pinch of grated nutmeg 3 ½ cups beef stock 6 ounces Ricotta cheese 1/2 cup double cream 1/3 cup parsley, roughly chopped

Directions

Press the "Sauté" button to heat up the Instant Pot. Once hot, cook the bacon until crisp; crumble with a fork and set aside. Now, brown the pork stew meat for 2 to 4 minutes, stirring frequently; set aside. Melt the butter; cook the onion and celery until softened. After that, add the garlic and sliced mushrooms; sauté until fragrant. Add all seasonings and beef stock. Return the reserved pork to the Instant Pot. Secure the lid. Choose the "Manual" setting and cook for 8 minutes at High pressure. Once cooking is complete, use a quick pressure release; carefully remove the lid. Afterwards, add Ricotta cheese, cream and parsley. Cover with the lid and allow it to sit for 15 minutes. Top with reserved bacon and enjoy!

Peperonata with Pork Sausages
(Ready in about 15 minutes | Servings 4)
Per serving: 582 Calories; 49.3g Fat; 9.1g Carbs; 24.5g Protein; 2.4g Sugars
Ingredients
1 teaspoon olive oil 8 pork sausages, casing removed 1 green bell pepper, seeded and sliced 1 red bell pepper, seeded and sliced 1 jalapeño pepper, seeded and sliced 1 red onion, chopped 2 garlic cloves, minced 2 Roma tomatoes, puréed 1 cup roasted vegetable broth 1 tablespoon Italian seasoning 2 tablespoons fresh Italian parsley 2 tablespoons ripe olives, pitted and sliced
Directions Press the "Sauté" button to heat up the Instant Pot. Once hot, add the oil; sear your sausages until no longer pink in center. Add the other ingredients, except for the olives and parsley; stir to combine well. Secure the lid. Choose the "Manual" setting and cook for 8 minutes at High pressure. Once cooking is complete, use a quick pressure release; carefully remove the lid. Serve garnished with fresh parsley and olives. Bon appétit!

Noodle-less Classic Lasagna
(Ready in about 20 minutes | Servings 6)
Per serving: 539 Calories; 41.1g Fat; 5g Carbs; 36.2g Protein; 2.6g Sugars
Ingredients
1 tablespoon olive oil 1 1/3 pounds ground pork 1 teaspoon garlic, finely minced 2 tablespoons scallions, finely chopped 1 teaspoon dried oregano 1 teaspoon dried basil 1/2 teaspoon dried rosemary 20 ounces pasta sauce, sugar-free 1 cup cream cheese 1 cup Romano cheese 2 eggs 6 ounces Swiss cheese, sliced
Directions
Press the "Sauté" button to heat up the Instant Pot. Heat the olive oil and cook the ground meat with the garlic and scallions for 2 to 4 minutes, stirring continuously. Add oregano, basil, rosemary, and pasta sauce. Now, add 1/2 of this meat sauce to a lightly greased baking dish. Then, in a mixing bowl, thoroughly combine the cream cheese, Romano cheese, and eggs. Place this cheese mixture over the meat layer. Add the remaining 1/2 of the meat mixture. Top with Swiss cheese. Cover with a sheet of aluminum foil and make a foil sling if needed. Add 1 ½ cups of water and metal rack to the Instant Pot. Lower the baking dish onto the metal rack. Secure the lid. Choose the "Manual" setting and cook for 9 minutes at High pressure. Once cooking is complete, use a quick pressure release; carefully remove the lid. Bon appétit!

Pork Tenderloin "Rosa di Parma"
(Ready in about 1 hour 20 minutes | Servings 4
Per serving: 333 Calories; 17.6g Fat; 4.1g Carbs; 38g Protein; 0.5g Sugars
Ingredients
4 pork tenderloins, butterflied 1/2 teaspoon ground black pepper 1/2 teaspoon cayenne pepper Sea salt, to taste 1/2 cup leeks, sliced 1 cup vegetable broth 1 tablespoon olive oil 1 tablespoon rice wine 2 tablespoons coconut aminos 1 teaspoon fresh sage, chopped 4 slices Italian Parma ham 1/2 cup Parmigiano-Reggiano cheese, freshly grated 2 tablespoons butter, divided
Directions
Season the pork tenderloins with black pepper, cayenne pepper, and sea salt. In a mixing bowl, thoroughly combine the leeks, broth, olive oil, wine, coconut aminos, and sage. Add pork tenderloin and let it marinate at least 1 hour. Now, place the ham slices on the tenderloins. Divide Parmigiano-Reggiano cheese among pork tenderloins. Then, tightly roll up each tenderloin. Secure with the toothpicks. Press the "Sauté" button to heat up the Instant Pot. Melt the butter and sear tenderloins until delicately browned on both sides. Add the marinade and secure the lid. Choose the "Manual" setting and cook for 12 minutes at High pressure. Once cooking is complete, use a quick pressure release; carefully remove the lid. Bon appétit!

Cheesy Salsa Meatloaf

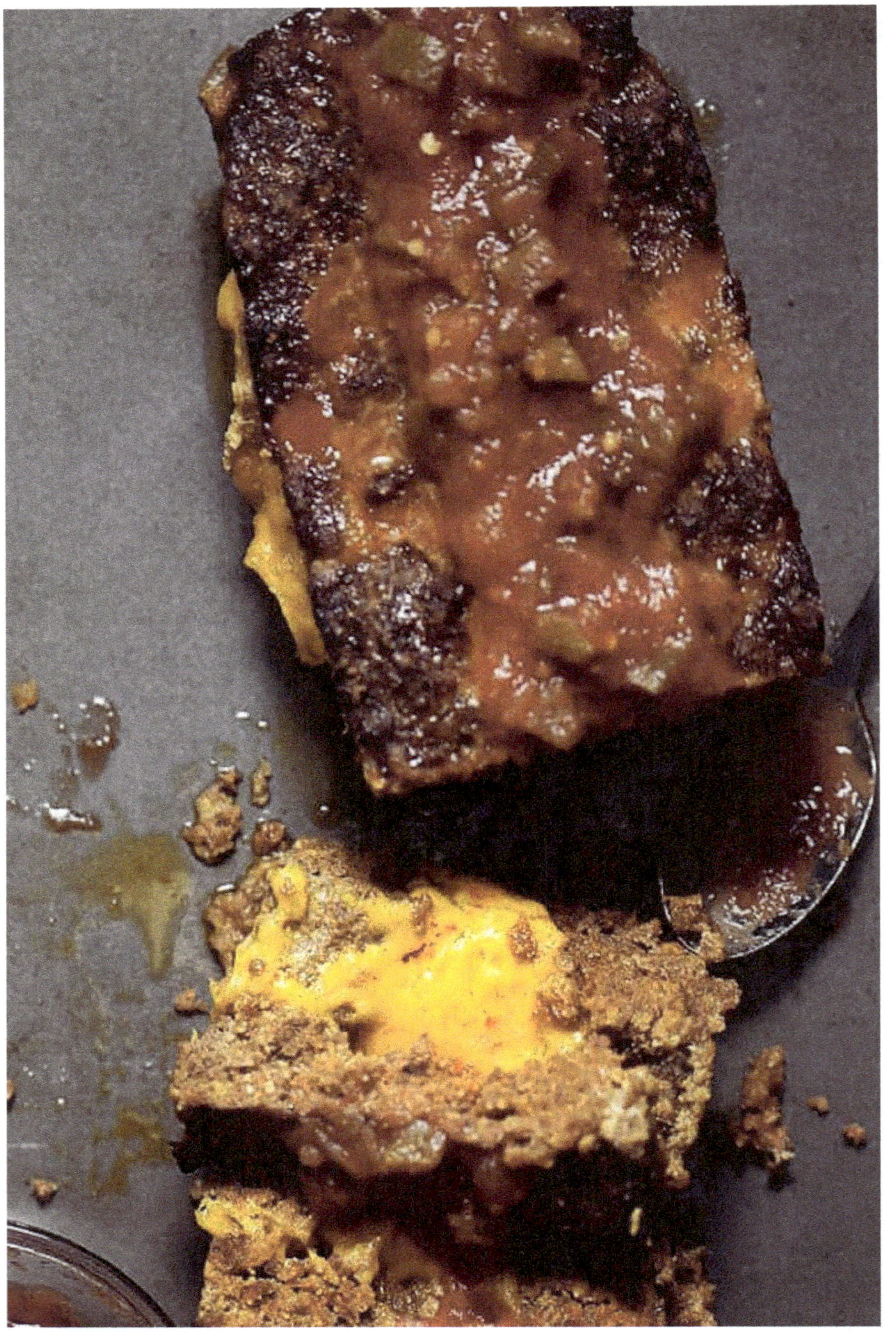

(Ready in about 35 minutes | Servings 6)

Per serving: 468 Calories; 35.7g Fat; 1.6g Carbs; 33.6g Protein; 1.2g Sugars

Ingredients

1 ½ pounds ground pork 1/2 pound ground chuck 1/2 teaspoon sea salt 1/2 teaspoon ground black pepper 1 teaspoon red pepper flakes, crushed 1/2 teaspoon ground bay leaf 1 teaspoon brown mustard 2 eggs, whisked 2/3 cup cream cheese 6 thin slices bacon 1/3 cup tomatillo salsa

Directions Prepare your Instant Pot by adding 1 ½ cups of water and metal rack to the bottom of the inner pot. In a mixing dish, thoroughly combine ground meat, salt, black pepper, red pepper flakes, ground bay leaf, brown mustard, eggs, and cream cheese. Shape the mixture into the meatloaf. Place the meatloaf in a baking pan. Now, arrange bacon slices, crosswise over meatloaf, overlapping them slightly. Top with tomatillo salsa. Secure the lid. Choose the "Manual" setting and cook for 30 minutes at High pressure. Once cooking is complete, use a quick pressure release; carefully remove the lid. Enjoy!

Tamarind Pork Spare Ribs
(Ready in about 25 minutes | Servings 4
Per serving: 266 Calories; 9.7g Fat; 6.2g Carbs; 36.7g Protein; 2.9g Sugars
Ingredients
1 ½ pounds spare ribs 1 thin sliced fresh ginger, peeled 4 garlic cloves, halved 1 jalapeño pepper, thinly sliced 1 bay leaf 1/2 teaspoon black peppercorns 1 tablespoon tamarind paste 1 teaspoon shrimp paste Sea salt and ground black pepper, to taste 1/2 cup marinara sauce
Directions
Arrange spare ribs on the bottom of your Instant Pot. Add fresh ginger, garlic, jalapeño pepper, bay leaf, and peppercorns. Next, mix the tamarind paste, shrimp paste, salt, black pepper, marinara sauce, and water. Pour this tamarind sauce over the ribs in the Instant Pot. Add enough water to cover the spare ribs. Secure the lid. Choose the "Manual" setting and cook for 20 minutes at High pressure. Once cooking is complete, use a quick pressure release; carefully remove the lid. Serve warm and enjoy!

Ground Pork Taco Casserole

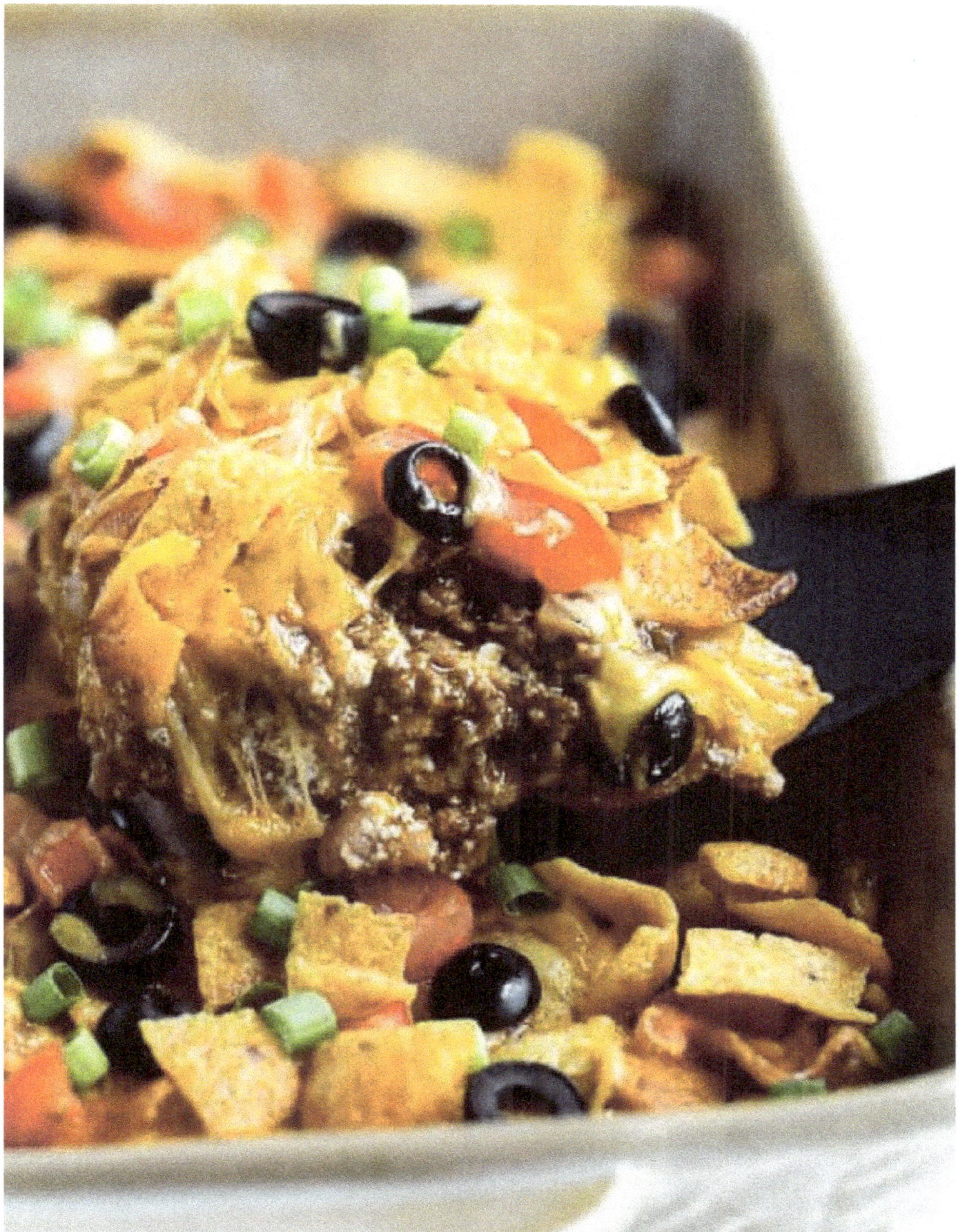

(Ready in about 35 minutes | Servings 6)
Per serving: 409 Calories; 31.6g Fat; 4.7g Carbs; 25.7g Protein; 2.7g Sugars

Ingredients

3 ounces Cottage cheese, at room temperature 1/4 cup double cream 2 eggs 1 teaspoon taco seasoning 6 ounces Cotija cheese, crumbled 3/4 pound ground pork 1 tablespoon taco seasoning 1/2 cup tomatoes, puréed 3 ounces chopped green chilies 6 ounces Queso Manchego cheese, shredded

Directions

Prepare your Instant Pot by adding 1 ½ cups of water and a metal rack to the bottom of the inner pot. In a mixing bowl, thoroughly combine Cottage cheese, double cream, eggs, and taco seasoning. Lightly grease a casserole dish; spread the Cotija cheese over the bottom. Pour in the Cottage/ egg mixture as evenly as possible. Lower the casserole dish onto the rack. Secure the lid. Choose "Manual" mode and High pressure; cook for 20 minutes. Once cooking is complete, use a quick pressure release; carefully remove the lid. In the meantime, heat a cast-iron skillet over a moderately high heat. Now, brown ground pork, crumbling it with a fork. Add taco seasoning, tomato purée and green chilies. Spread this mixture over the prepared cheese crust. Top with shredded Queso Manchego. Secure the lid. Choose "Manual" mode and High pressure; cook for 10 minutes. Once cooking is complete, use a quick pressure release; carefully remove the lid. Serve and enjoy!

CPSIA information can be obtained
at www.ICGtesting.com
Printed in the USA
LVHW061737250521
688475LV00012B/856

9 781008 9535